# THE TRAUMA OF CAPTIVITY

# THE TRAUMA OF CAPTIVITY

POW Mental Health – What Happened When Soldiers Returned Home

**JULIE COOK**

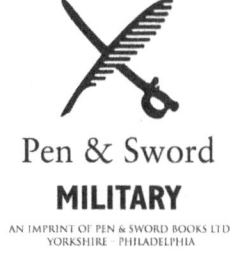

Pen & Sword
**MILITARY**
AN IMPRINT OF PEN & SWORD BOOKS LTD.
YORKSHIRE – PHILADELPHIA

First published in Great Britain in 2023 by
PEN AND SWORD MILITARY
An imprint of
Pen & Sword Books Limited
Yorkshire – Philadelphia

Copyright © Julie Cook, 2023

ISBN 978 1 39901 682 7

The right of Julie Cook to be identified as Author of this work has been asserted by her in accordance with the Copyright, Designs and Patents Act 1988.

A CIP catalogue record for this book is available from the British Library.

All rights reserved. No part of this book may be reproduced or transmitted in any form or by any means, electronic or mechanical including photocopying, recording or by any information storage and retrieval system, without permission from the Publisher in writing.

Typeset in Times New Roman 12/16 by
SJmagic DESIGN SERVICES, India.
Printed and bound in the UK by CPI Group (UK) Ltd.

Pen & Sword Books Limited incorporates the imprints of Atlas, Archaeology, Aviation, Discovery, Family History, Fiction, History, Maritime, Military, Military Classics, Politics, Select, Transport, True Crime, Air World, Frontline Publishing, Leo Cooper, Remember When, Seaforth Publishing, The Praetorian Press, Wharncliffe Local History, Wharncliffe Transport, Wharncliffe True Crime and White Owl.

*For a complete list of Pen & Sword titles please contact*
PEN & SWORD BOOKS LIMITED
George House, Units 12 & 13, Beevor Street, Off Pontefract Road,
Barnsley, South Yorkshire, S71 1HN, England
E-mail: enquiries@pen-and-sword.co.uk
Website: www.pen-and-sword.co.uk

or

PEN AND SWORD BOOKS
1950 Lawrence Rd, Havertown, PA 19083, USA
E-mail: uspen-and-sword@casematepublishers.com
Website: www.penandswordbooks.com

# Contents

| | | |
|---|---|---|
| Acknowledgements | | vi |
| Introduction | | vii |
| Chapter One | Man strays onto battlefield | 1 |
| Chapter Two | The First World War: 'While of unsound mind…' | 15 |
| Chapter Three | Psychological Intervention | 39 |
| Chapter Four | Prisoners of War in Germany – Second World War | 58 |
| Chapter Five | Japan and the Far East | 88 |
| Chapter Six | Coming home from Japan: Compensation and carrying on | 117 |
| Chapter Seven | Glorification versus Reality | 144 |
| Notes | | 169 |
| Bibliography | | 175 |

# Acknowledgements

I wish to thank the following people who have helped me in the researching of this book: Howard Georgia Fitz-Gerald for pointing me in the direction of some good prisoner of war social media groups, authors Michelle Rawlins and Kate Thompson. Thanks to Jonathan Wright, Commissioning Editor at Pen and Sword Military for commissioning this work. Thanks to Karyn Burnham copy editor. To Stephen Noble at the Red Cross archives who was so kind as to source specific documents for me. Thank you to the amazing charity COFEPOW, the charity that keeps Far East POWs' memories alive, and Chris Wills their events coordinator for putting me in touch with so many prisoner of war family members. Thanks to the British Newspaper Archive for their incredible wealth of articles regarding prisoners of war during both world wars.

A huge thank you to Gulf War POW fast jet RAF pilot John Peters for his reflections on his time as a prisoner of war in Iraq. Finally, and most importantly, a sincere thank you to the sons and daughters of prisoners of war who were generous enough to share the stories of their fathers with me: Mandy Procter, Margaret Kiernan, Lorna Doyle, Dave Clarke, David Reader, Kevin Goodwin, Chris Ramsbottom. Their stories are moving, emotional and, in some cases, heart-breaking and also include tales of great bravery and endurance.

These stories will ensure their fathers' memories live on.

# Introduction

The idea for this book began in tiny seed form when I re-read my great-grandfather David Parker's war diaries. He was a prisoner of war in Germany during the First World War. His war story, like so many, was a harrowing one.

He'd been called up. He was not a career soldier, but a normal family man from Lancashire. Thrown into the Belgian theatre of the First World War, he fought hand-to-hand with a German soldier before being bayoneted through the head. He should have died. Instead, he woke up and found himself in a Belgian convent-hospital being treated by nuns. Many men might have felt relief, both at being alive and being removed from the danger of the battlefield. But that was not the end of Private Parker's war story. During his recovery, the hospital was stormed by German troops and he and the other patients were taken as prisoners of war.

While he was prisoner, he started to write diaries. The diaries – written in flowing, beautiful cursive handwriting – look nothing special at first. They are written in two small, lined exercise books; the sort you have at school. When I was a child, these books were kept safely in a protective bag on a bookshelf. When I first discovered them, I asked again and again to read them but was told they might be too upsetting. 'When you're older,' was the refrain.

When I finally did read them as a teenager I was in awe, not only of all my great-grandfather had gone through (fighting in the trenches with no previous soldiering experience, surviving being bayoneted, being taken prisoner, starved, hit, abused) but also of how 'normal' he was described as being when he came home.

My questions were the usual ones:

Was he violent? No.
Was he a heavy drinker? No.
Did he go off into prolonged silences? No.
Did he ever work again? Yes, for the rest of his life.

His diaries spoke of horrors, such as watching German soldiers crucifying an elderly Belgian farm owner trying to protect his home, of being starved, of beatings and unending forced labour in quarries. Yet, whenever I asked my maternal side of the family how he was on his return it was always the same response: fine.

It made me question just what it was like for prisoners of war when they returned home. How did they adapt from going from an ordinary husband, son or brother, to a fighter and then a prisoner and then back again? How did they resettle back into society after the war?

What was offered to them by way of help? Mental health is a relatively modern term – what was the treatment for men who suffered mentally after being a POW in the last century?

I then began researching more and asked myself questions. What does being a prisoner of war mean? What emotions does the term evoke? Bravery? Despair? Sorrow? Hardship? Violence? Starvation? Abuse? Camaraderie? Wish to escape?

Many of us can only guess at what it might have been like to be a POW from our own cultural references, from films or books. It is true that being a prisoner of war has been dramatised countless times over the decades. The camaraderie, the bravery, the ill-treatment, the despair and hope: there is something about watching a band of brothers held captive that appeals to our innermost psyche. There is no surprise that POW films have been some of the most successful

# INTRODUCTION

productions in history, winners of Oscars, repeated on television for decades to come.

*The Bridge on the River Kwai* showed the hardships of being a prisoner of war. It won seven Oscars and is still referred to as one of the greatest films of all time. *The Great Escape*, starring Steve McQueen and Richard Attenborough, told of the bravery and pluck of those who dared to flee and now has one of the most famous theme tunes of all time, often played irreverently at football matches.

Over the years since the two great wars, we have glorified what it meant to be a prisoner of war. We have made these prisoners' stories part of our own cultural reference points about what it means to be British, what it means to be a soldier, what it means to be on one side and not another. But while these films are important pieces of cultural history, they may have inadvertently contributed to a collective 'glossing over' of the unspeakable realities of being a prisoner of war. With their healthy-looking actors, fighting spirit that never seemed to cease, upbeat theme music accompanying their every manoeuvre, did these films tell the truth about what life was like as a prisoner of war? Or have they made many of us believe that being a prisoner of war was a game of eluding captors, of plucky British humour and positivity?

It is not only films, of course. There are thousands upon thousands of books about prisoners of war – this book one of them. Some are written by the hand of prisoners of war themselves, others from historians and military experts. Prisoners of war stories evoke sympathy, national pride and jingoism.

As for jingoism and prisoner of war representations, many of the family members of prisoners of war I interviewed for this book said their relatives had mixed feelings about our most famous POW films and our attitudes to what it meant to be a prisoner in wartime. Some of their relatives could not stand to watch such films. Others found them amusing because they were so far from what their lives as prisoners of war had been. Others simply said the films did not give an accurate representation at all so were of no import to the returning soldiers.

# THE TRAUMA OF CAPTIVITY

But it is not just how prisoners of war were treated in the camps that have been misrepresented over the years. There is a gaping hole in our histories as to how those men fared when they returned home. What happened when they put down their rifles, took off their Army-issue combats and sat down to breakfast with their wives and children? How did they adapt? Did they talk about what they went through? Or did they bury the terrors and horrors they had seen?

The imprisonment for many POWs did not end when they were set free or escaped. Many psychiatrists and psychologists examined returning prisoners of war after their repatriation and found that their sense of imprisonment lingered, long after they stepped foot again on British soil. Some psychological studies from the time assured readers that the neurotic traits displayed by returning prisoners of war would only 'last six months'. Others claimed that many of the neuroses of returning POWs were not, in fact, due to their imprisonment abroad but were caused by early childhood experiences, a lack of a father, lack of discipline and delinquency. Were these psychological studies simply a reflection of the time and the 1940s and 1950s attitudes towards mental health?

In my interviews with the sons and daughters of ex-prisoners of war for this book, many said their father never did recover fully. Others I interviewed, by contrast, said their father never displayed any change in character. So, did it depend on just that – character? Could two men go through the same ordeal as a prisoner of war and one return damaged and traumatised, the other healthy in mind and able to carry on as before? Some psychological studies, often of hundreds of returning soldiers, claimed that a soldier's upbringing and early childhood neuroses would influence how he was affected by imprisonment. Was this the powers that be holding their hands up and denying all responsibility for how a man reacted after being imprisoned? Was it not the 'fault' of the war at all, but merely a question of character?

# INTRODUCTION

Another important question to consider when examining returning prisoners of war is that of rank and class. It is of no doubt that the average foot soldier had a very different experience in both war and imprisonment than an officer. In many German camps, foot soldiers did the work and officers had a very different experience, often sleeping on beds rather than heaps of straw as their inferiors did. Did class, therefore, affect not only how a prisoner of war endured his time in a prison camp, but also have an effect on how his return to normal life would play out?

From an economic point of view, it would no doubt be easier for a returning officer prisoner to be housed, clothed and have enough finances to survive, than a returning lower-rank soldier prisoner who would have to worry about finding lodgings, work and so on. This in mind, this book will look at the importance of associations, groups and clubs for returning working-class prisoners of war, to be able to find other like-minded men who had gone through the same ordeal, and of the same class.

Clubs and associations were set up – and many, like the incredible FEPOW (Far East Prisoners of War) still help families of prisoners of war today. CRUs – civil resettlement units – were also of huge importance and support to returning prisoners of war. They were a place where prisoners could reassess, regroup, and stay until they felt ready to face their reality once again after repatriation. They realised early on that 'hutted camps' would be too similar to the accommodation the prisoners had lived in during their incarceration and so often the CRUs were held in more welcoming settings – in recommissioned stately homes and other country houses – to allow the soldiers to recuperate in more luxurious surroundings than those they had endured abroad.

But while the government, the Ministry of Defence, renowned psychologists and charities and individuals did their best to ensure returning prisoners of war got the treatment they needed, what happened when those men returned to family life? What happened behind closed doors, over the kitchen table, in the workplace, or when disciplining children? How did a man's experience of being a prisoner of war affect him as a husband, a worker and a father? This book will of course cover what life as a prisoner of war was like, but its aim is to examine what happened to prisoners of war when their captivity ended. It will ask how they were supported on their return home, how they managed financially, emotionally, physically and mentally.

Mental health as we know it today was not discussed in such depth or as frequently after the two world wars. In the First World War, 'shell-shock' was the closest that terminology came to addressing mental health concerns – and even that was open to debate in the months after the war. It is also worth considering whether, in a war where so many men did not return home, there was any place for those who had been prisoners to complain openly or wished to discuss their feelings?

As for the Second World War, prisoners of war who had been held in Germany and the Far East, on the most part, were expected to return home and resume life where they had left it. They would become husbands to wives they had not seen in years, sons to parents who had yearned to hear from them, fathers once again to children they barely knew and might have changed beyond recognition while they were away. They would need to find work and provide for their families again. But what was it like for them returning to this normal world? In a world where little was known about post-traumatic stress, depression and anxiety – how did these men learn to live again in normal civilian life?

Some First and Second World War psychiatrists and psychologists pushed the idea that fresh air and exercise could 'cure' men of any neuroses after being held captive. In more distressing situations, other experts of the time believed that exposing the returning prisoner to his fear was the best way for him to recover – for example, exposing the returning POW afraid of enclosed spaces to more enclosed spaces;

## INTRODUCTION

placing a man afraid of loud noises from war on the front-facing busy road of a hospital, and so on. Others believed that the 'six-month' average length of such neuroses were of no cause for concern and believed concern was only necessary when a man complained of symptoms of nerves, irritability, violence, alcoholism or stress after the six months had passed. This made it incredibly difficult for family members of returning POWs to know what was normal and what was not, what was acceptable and what was not and – most importantly – when to seek help.

If a POW hit his wife in the first six months after returning, was this to be expected and should be forgiven? If a POW could not stand to be out of doors for more than six months after his return, when should a family seek help – and how? This mix of responses from psychologists, doctors, psychiatrists and people in government meant that for many years many families suffered irreparable damage to their relationships. In this book I speak to daughters whose fathers could never hug them again, or even speak properly to them. I hear of mothers who were treated badly by a returning husband after his incarceration and of the affect this had on children's mental health for years to come.

Then there is the anger. Former Japanese prisoners of war fought for fifty years to get compensation for the cruelty they had endured. Finally, in 2000, relatives of those who had been held prisoner in the Far East camps were awarded a one-off payment of £10,000. The government said the tax-free payment would repay a debt of honour owed to British POWs who had thus far been 'forgotten people', and sent the awards to 16,700 people which included more than 4,500 widows. Over 50,000 British troops – and civilians – were captured in Singapore and 25 per cent died, so for many this compensation was too little, too late. By 2000 many of the prisoners of war had died, never receiving their compensation. Many of their widows had died too, leaving only their children behind to receive the awards. Many of these grown-up children were angered at the small sum of £10,000 which was supposed to cover a lifetime of stomach problems, dysentery, worms, bone problems, vitamin B insufficiency from starvation and, of course, the mental health damage borne from a regime of incomprehensible cruelty.

A sum of £10,000 might have helped fifty years earlier, some argued, but not now that their fathers and mothers had had to live with a lifetime of pain and suffering as well as feeling 'forgotten' by the world for what they had gone through. With the help of those same sons and daughters of ex-prisoners of war, and diaries and interviews from prisoners themselves, this book aims to answer the question: after the trauma of captivity, what happened when soldiers returned home?

# Chapter One

# Man strays onto battlefield

'Prisoners of war are in the power of the hostile government, but not of the individuals or corps who capture them. They must be humanely treated. All their personal belongings, except arms, horses, and military papers, remain their property.'

*Hague Convention IV, 1907*

'What a nation you are! You fight like lions, and once you have beaten your enemies you treat them as though they were your best friends!'

General von Salm, taken from *A Memory of Solferino*

While other young men of the time were saying goodbye to their families and setting off on the ubiquitous European Grand Tour to Venice or Paris, one man chose not to. His name was Henry Dunant. While his peers might have been embarking on journeys of artistic and sexual self-discovery across the capital cities of Europe, Dunant stayed home in his native Switzerland and joined the Geneva Society for Alms Giving. He did not know it then, but in time he would become a name synonymous with equality and brotherhood, with seeing past the sides of war and treating all – enemy, adversary, prisoner – with the same fairness. He would become an advocate for treating prisoners of war as those who held them would wish to be treated.

# THE TRAUMA OF CAPTIVITY

Dunant was born in Geneva in 1828 to religious parents who performed benevolent social work like other families held tea parties. Their Christian charity rubbed off on the young Henry and he grew into a caring, politically and socially-conscious young man, full of ideas to change the world. In his early twenties he founded the Geneva section of the YMCA, and a year later he toured Algeria, Tunisia and Sicily and wrote a book about his experiences.

Dunant lived in an era of great upheaval. He had lived to hear and read about the Crimean war, during which 900,000 soldiers had died. Crimea was one of the first wars to be widely documented in journalism, newspapers and photographs, as well as one of the first to use modern warfare in which technology won out over soldierly tactics. Dunant was a contemporary and admirer of Florence Nightingale (she was eight years his senior). And while her pioneering work at Scutari to change the way hospitals and nursing was seen forever, inspired by her desire to alleviate suffering in war, she would, in time, disagree with Dunant's future ideas on neutrality.

But that was in the future. Dunant was not only a Christian thinker but also a businessman like his father before him, and he started a trading company called the société financière et industrielle des Moulins des Mons-Djémila. He planned to grow corn but his plans were scuppered when local authorities were not supportive and water rights were in doubt. So, the young Dunant had to appeal to the highest echelons in charge of the region: namely Emperor Napoleon III.

Napoleon III was nephew of Napoleon himself and his headquarters at that time were in Solferino, a town in what would become a part of Italy when its regions later joined. Durant needed Napoleon III to put in a good word with the colonial powers that be in the regions where he wanted to start his corn growing business, and so he wrote flattering prose about Napoleon III before travelling to Solferino to meet him.

He arrived on 24 June 1859. As fate would have it, the date was the same day a battle between the alliance of the French and Piedmont-Sardinian army against the Austrian had taken place. As Dunant arrived,

## MAN STRAYS ONTO BATTLEFIELD

exhausted from his journey, he met people who lived locally; stunned, they talked in hushed tones of the battle that had ensued that day. The battle had ceased now. The guns no longer fired. But Dunant felt compelled to view the battlefield for himself, to see what had happened.

When he arrived at the land between the villages of Solferino and San Martino, just south of Lake Garda, he saw scenes that would alter the course of his life and career. That day, while he had been travelling to meet Napoleon III, 230,000 men had fought in battle for twelve hours, often in chaotic, hand-to-hand combat. As a result, now, hours later, 23,000 men lay wounded and dying on the battlefield.

Quite by chance, Dunant found himself in the middle of hell. It was true he had not witnessed the battle itself, but the horror of it endured. Now he made his way to the battlefield, compelled to walk among the dead and dying, hearing their groans of agony, their pleas of help, their desperate requests to be dispatched humanely. Staggering through the horror, Dunant found himself in numb shock at how little care there was now for the dying. He'd gone from his frustrated plans to begin his corn business, to stepping over groaning, twisted bodies. To his shock, there were no orderlies taking the dying away, no medics to ease their pain in their final throes. There was no water for the thirsty. No medical supplies. Battle had been fought. Enemy had fought enemy. But in the end, when death the equaliser knocked all down, there was no last humanity for these soldiers in their final moments. He wrote:

> From the midst of all this fighting, which went on and on all over the battlefield, arose the oaths and curses of men of all the different nations engaged – men, of whom many had been made into murderers at the age of twenty![1]

Something kicked the stunned man into action and, forgetting momentarily his business plans, he used his natural organisation skills and gathered locals together, telling others to knock on doors, bringing men, women and girls together to help the wounded soldiers. He donated his own money to buy medicines, bandages and the materials to erect on-the-spot battlefield hospital tents. He watched as soldiers were carried off and saw horrific operations to save lives involving nothing more than a saw and a piece of cloth clenched between the teeth for gangrenous limbs. He saw wounded men turn into boys again, begging for their mothers. He helped comrades find each other. He was practical, quick-thinking.

But most importantly, he took *no side.*

Despite this instinct to be proactive and practical, the horrors of what Dunant saw never left him. He wrote them down – with graphic, horrific detail – and personally paid for 1,600 copies to be printed and distributed. These memories, he hoped, would stir people into action in time for the 'next' war so that the horrors might not be repeated. What seems to have moved Dunant the most was that, after the battle was over, soldiers became 'human' once again, looking for their friends, searching desperately for comrades.

> Towards the end of the day, when the shades of night began to cover this immense field of slaughter, many a French officer and soldier went searching high and low for a comrade, a countryman, or a friend. If he came across someone he knew, he would kneel at his side trying to bring him back to life, press his hand, staunch the bleeding, or bind the broken limb with a handkerchief. But there was no water to be had for the poor sufferer. How many silent tears were shed that miserable night when all false pride, all human even, were forgotten?[2]

Dunant does not hold back in his prose. His is not a book about heroism (although he does touch on individual heroic acts), but a book about the futility of war, of how 'the stillness of the night was broken by groans, by stifled sighs of anguish and suffering. Heartrending voices kept calling for help. Who could ever describe the agonies of that fearful night?'[3]

As he had stepped over the dead and the dying, Dunant was met with horrors he would never forget. Some soldiers, he recalled, had a calm expression, while others were 'disfigured by the torments of their death-struggle', while others' hands were 'clawing at the ground, their eyes staring wildly, their moustaches bristling above clenched teeth that were bared in a sinister convulsive grin.'[4]

Interestingly, Dunant writes not only about the last throes of the dying but also remarks on how each side dealt with its prisoners. In a world and a time where there were no rules on how prisoners of war should be treated, Dunant noted that it varied wildly depending on who was taking whom.

> Some French soldiers were minded to take reprisals on a few prisoners whom they took for Croats, saying angrily that 'those tight-trousers', as they call them, always killed the wounded. The prisoners were in reality Hungarians who wear a uniform similar to that of the Croats but are much less cruel. I succeeded in explaining this distinction to the French soldiers and in getting the trembling Hungarians away from them. However for the most part, with very few exceptions, the feeling of the French towards their prisoners was nothing but goodwill.[5]

But for German prisoners of war, Dunant was worried as these men were:

> forced to suffer not only physical pain, but also the griefs of captivity. And now they must endure the ill will of the Milanese who have a profound hatred for their race, for their leaders, and for their sovereign. These men could count on little sympathy until they should reach French

soil. Ah poor mothers in Germany, in Austria, in Hungary and Bohemia, how can one help thinking of their agony, when they hear that their sons are wounded and prisoners in this hostile land![6]

The notion that prisoners should be treated equally, just as the dead or dying should once battle was over, is something that is profoundly clear in Dunant's work. He makes no comment on who is to blame, or whose side is 'right' or who is wrong. He writes solely of how soldiers and prisoners of war, after battle, should be equal and treated as such. He moved among the local people and, showing them his belief that soldiers should be treated with kindness and sympathy no matter what their side, he found that they quickly followed his example. Many local women who agreed to volunteer as nurses and orderlies called out: '*Tutti Fratelli*!' – all are brothers – to which Dunant replied: 'All honour to these compassionate women, to these girls of Castiglione!'[7]

It is true that Dunant's book is a harrowing read. The descriptions of the twisted corpses, the injured young men begging to be killed quickly and allowed to die, the crying boys who only wanted to see their mother again, cannot fail to move the hardest reader. But like all good writers, Dunant was using this horror as a catalyst for action. It was a political work. He wanted things to change:

> But why have I told of all these scenes of pain and distress, and perhaps aroused painful emotions in my readers? Why have I lingered with seeming complacency over lamentable pictures, tracing their details with what may appear desperate fidelity? It is a natural question. Perhaps I might answer it by another: Would it not be possible, in time of peace and quiet, to form relief societies for the purpose of having care given to the wounded in wartime by zealous, devoted, and thoroughly qualified volunteers?[8]

## MAN STRAYS ONTO BATTLEFIELD

Returning from the horrors he had seen, Henry Dunant was unable to escape the idea that more should be done for soldiers both during and after battle and when they were taken prisoner. He saw that soldiers, on the whole, wanted to aid one another. He saw enemies bandage each other up when they were wounded, he saw French soldiers carry Austrian soldiers on their backs to their camp when they needed medical care. His words '*tutti fratelli*' were simple but yet so obvious. Soldiers, to his mind, were all equal on the battlefield. After that battle, equality should remain. Treatment of the wounded should be given, regardless of side or nationality. Prisoners should be treated with respect and goodwill despite the hatred of those who had captured them.

An idea took shape in his mind, the idea of a future neutral organisation that should be created to give care to wounded soldiers – without reference to what side they were fighting for. His book was distributed around Europe to political leaders and military men. One man who received a copy was Gustave Moynier, then the president of the Geneva Society for Public Welfare. When the organisation held its meeting in 1863, Moynier referred to Dunant's book and the members at his meeting were receptive, so much so that a five-person committee was formed to assess Dunant's proposals further. The main points Dunant wanted to be implemented were respect and care to be given to soldiers regardless of the side they were on, and medical treatment to be given on the battlefield without fear of volunteers being attacked.

Two weeks later, on 17 February 1863, the committee met again and included Moynier, two doctors, Swiss Army General Henri Dufour with the final member being Dunant himself. They did not know it, of course, but this day would become known as the founding of the ICRC – the International Committee of the Red Cross. Based on the notion that soldiers should not only be treated with humanity, but also that this should be irrespective of which side they had fought for, Dunant's ideas were ground-breaking for their day. Until this point soldiers in war were, arguably, seen just as in the Latin origin of their name 'soldarius', meaning a man 'having pay'.

It is believed that organised warfare began around 3000 BC and the first 'standing army' is thought to have been created around 2250 bc by Sargon of Agade. His army is thought to have been made up of 100,000 paid soldiers, with specialist units such as cavalry and bowmen. Great interest was put into making the soldier – no matter what era he happened to be fighting in – into the greatest machine of war. Trained in weaponry (swords or, later, guns), trained in close combat, trained in attack and defence. And of course, at no point in this early history was any thought given to a soldier's mental health. In the grand scheme of things, 'mental health' is a phrase that has only just arrived.

A soldier would have been elevated above normal male society. Stronger, bigger, better, harder, more able. *Paid.* While others bartered or traded, soldiers were the first to receive income for doing something other than what their fathers or forefathers had done. For aeons, having pay for being a mercenary fighter had left soldiers on the outside of humanity, revered for bravery but dismissed, perhaps, as undeserving of care or sympathy or aid when a battle was over. The phrase 'soldier on' became synonymous with carrying on against adversity, putting up with things, hardening yourself.

For Dunant to propose the idea that mercenary soldiers should be treated with care when wounded or ailing, and given an immunity during that period of ailing, was seminal for the time. But not everyone agreed with him. Dunant pressed that at the heart of his idea to start an organisation was the notion of neutrality. Moynier, a pragmatist, had his concerns. He said that neutrality was not only unfeasible but unthinkable in times of war when hatred and jingoism ran deep. However, in time Moynier – an evangelical Christian and charity worker within forty groups ranging from caring for orphans to working with prisoners – defined the idea of a new neutral service. It would be called the Red Cross – because its symbol would be a white flag with a red cross at its centre. This should be internationally recognised and therefore be neutral in times of war.

Moynier defined the principles of the Red Cross, saying that there could only be one Red Cross per country, that the societies must be ready at all times, that they must make preparations for war in times of peace, that they must have willingness to help all wounded and sick regardless of their nationality or side, and that the different Red Crosses from around the world should help each other. Moynier said that the International Red Cross should be 'the voluntary guardian of these Principles so crucial to our work'.

A rather famous contemporary of this was Florence Nightingale. She had returned from the Crimean war and had set up the Nightingale Training School at St Thomas's Hospital in London. If one woman understood soldiers' mental health it was her. In letters between Dunant and Nightingale, she argued that the governments of opposing warring countries should make it their duty to ensure their soldiers had adequate aid, medical supplies, and that providing a neutral organisation such as the Red Cross would be to allow such governments to wash their hands of their responsibility. Eight months later, however, in October 1863, fourteen states attended a meeting in Geneva to discuss the care of wounded soldiers. A year later, in summer 1864, a diplomatic conference was held by the neutral Swiss government where the First Geneva Convention was signed by twelve states. The agreements reached at the convention included: relief to the wounded without any distinction to nationality, neutrality of medical personnel, a distinctive red cross sign on a white background.

But intentions, however good, did not last long. In 1870 Prussian forces marched on Paris during the Franco-Prussian war and took the city; 400 were killed after a twenty-three-night bombardment. Those that weren't killed, were starved. A shortage of meat during the war meant that Parisians were eating dogs, cats and even rats. Even the city's only pair of elephants were slaughtered for meat. With such horrors occurring only a few years after the Geneva Convention had been signed, people wondered if there had been any point to it at all.

> Geneva Convention Doomed: The last sortie brought with it an increase in the odium which has fallen on the Geneva Convention by breaches of its rules and abuses of its privileges ... I am obliged to hear then, that when the attack on the posts near L'Hay and Chevilly on the 29th November had been made, ambulances were sent out on both sides to pick up the wounded. A German waggon was thus employed in undiscriminating charity, relieving French and Germans alike. The officers and men in charge of the party observed a large white flag with a red cross, the Geneva Convention standard, flying outside an earthwork, one of the redoubt angels of Villejuif, where the French had planted it. They approached, gleaning as they went after the death harvest. Suddenly the fort opened on them, and the French lining the parapets poured musketry fire upon them, and obliged the whole ambulance to fly, not without causing loss. Again, there can be no doubt that the French took all the Bavarian and Prussian sick and wounded in the hospitals of Orleans and treated them as prisoners of war.[9]

It was perhaps becoming apparent that it was all too easy to set rules and dictats for opposing forces in the peaceful environs of a book-lined study over a mahogany table, but quite different when facing your enemy across a battlefield. Could the Geneva Convention work in practise as well as theory? Could it really endure the hatred that soldiers on opposing sides are taught to feel for their adversary? Could Dunant's notion of '*tutti fratelli*' really endure?

Later conventions were held and one took place at The Hague on 18 October 1907. On the topic of prisoners of war, it was decided that:

'Prisoners of War are in the power of the hostile government but not of the individuals or corps who capture them. They must be humanely treated. All their personal belongings, except arms, horses and military papers, remain their property.'[10] Prisoners of war, it was argued, could well suffer more than a wounded man on a battlefield because they were now at the mercy of a hostile state. Now the Convention discussed where and how these men must be interned and another annex was added:

> Prisoners of war may be interned in a town, fortress or camp, or other place, and bound not to go beyond certain fixed limits; but they cannot be confined except as indispensable measure of safety and only while the circumstances which necessitate the measure continue to exist.[11]

With confinement and personal property of prisoners of war discussed and agreed upon, the next annex was a controversial one: how did the state use prisoners of war for labour? At what point did work end and enforced slavery begin? The conference members discussed this at length and agreed on a longer annex, stating:

> The State may utilise the labour of prisoners of war according to their rank and aptitude, officers excepted. The tasks shall not be excessive and shall have no connection with the operations of the war.
>
> Prisoners may be authorised to work for the public service, for private persons, or on their own account.
>
> Work done for the State is paid for at the rates in force for work of a similar kind done by soldiers of the national army, or, if there are none in force, at a rate according to the work executed.
>
> When the work is for other branches of the public service or for private persons the conditions are settled in agreement with the military authorities.

## THE TRAUMA OF CAPTIVITY

> The wages of the prisoners shall go towards improving their position, and the balance shall be paid them on their release, after deducting the cost of their maintenance.[12]

The annex that followed agreed that the government to whose hands the prisoners of war have fallen would be 'charged with their maintenance', and that in the absence of a special agreement between the two sides, prisoners of war should be treated 'as regards board, lodging, and clothing on the same footing as the troops of the government who captured them'.[13]

Future prisoners of war might later smirk at the genteel description of 'board and lodging' in enemy camps, but at this time of hope (and innocence?) before the First World War and its horrors, the members of the Convention conference really did believe in their annexes. They believed that men could put aside their differences, their long-born hatred, their desire for vengeance of comrades they had lost, on national pride, and all the other multitudes of emotion and feeling that make up a soldier. *They believed.*

Other annexes were added relating to escape. It can be argued that the number one desire of a prisoner of war, after perhaps the longing to see their loved one, is to escape their confines. It is as natural as a bird in a cage wanting to flee. Therefore, the Convention decreed an entire annex on escapees and agreed that escaped prisoners who are retaken before being able to rejoin their own army would indeed be liable to disciplinary punishment. However, they also concluded that prisoners who were taken prisoner again after escaping would 'not be liable to any punishment on account of the previous flight'.[14]

The Convention was important because it laid out the exact laws and expectations of the imprisoning state but it also humanised prisoners. Interestingly, the Convention also extended these laws to individuals who followed an army without being directly in it, such as newspaper correspondents, reporters and contractors who might also fall into enemy hands. Prior to the convention these would have been merely collateral damage. Now, they too would be entitled to be treated as prisoners of war, provided they were in possession of a certificate from the army they were with.[15]

Other annexes dealt with relief societies for prisoners of war, namely that they should be given every opportunity to carry out their humane tasks such as tending to the wounded, bringing in supplies and distributing food and water. Also it was decreed that presents and relief and letters for prisoners of war should be admitted free from import or other duties. Religion – something close to the Christian Henry Dunant and Moynier's hearts – was also discussed. The new rules stated that prisoners of war would enjoy complete liberty to exercise their religion which would include being able to attend services at whichever church they might belong to as long as they complied with the orders issued by military authorities.[16]

And of huge importance was this annex:

> After the conclusion of peace, the repatriation of prisoners of war shall be carried out as quickly as possible.[17]

Forty-four nations signed the 1907 Hague Convention with a whole chapter – chapter two – devoted solely to the treatment of prisoners of war. The Anglo-Boer War of 1899–1902 was still present in many people's minds and thousands of prisoners had died in concentration camps in South Africa as a result of a measles epidemic. In other areas of the theatre of the Boer War, captors had simply not known what to do with such vast numbers of prisoners taken and had shipped them 'overseas' rather than hold them in camps. Now, for the future, there would be strict rules of how prisoners should be treated, where they should be held, and what was expected of captors.

Was this the end of the maltreatment of the soldier prisoner? Did this mark a new era of hope, of equality and charity towards one's enemy once the battle was over? What these benevolent and charitable men could never have foreseen, however, was that war would evolve. Machine guns would replace pistols and the growing far reach of the media would mean that hatred would run deeper, a call to arms would spread faster, and a war that no one could ever have imagined was just seven years away.

Could these laws stand the test of time? And could they be respected in a war that would end all wars?

As Dunant wrote in the final page of his book A Memory of Solferino:

> in an age when we hear so much of progress and civilisation, is it not a matter of urgency, since unhappily we cannot always avoid wars, to press forward in a humane and truly civilised spirit the attempt to prevent, or at least alleviate, the horrors of war?[18]

Time would tell if his idea of a humane and civilised spirit in war would prevail after the assassination of the Archduke Franz Ferdinand on the 28 June, 1914.

# Chapter Two

# The First World War: 'While of unsound mind...'

'Dear old Joe – I am fed up with life in general. I am off. Give my apologies to the boys. Best regards to yourself.'

Suicide letter left by Lance Corporal G. Wingate, Military Police, Dover, 1925

If the Crimean theatre of war was horrific in its magnitude, it was about to be dwarfed by a war to end all wars. Men from all social classes volunteered to fight in the First World War – in fact, at first, the government could not keep up with just how many wanted to enlist. A mix of social, political and national feeling fuelled the desire for men to go to war. But as the great war poet Siegfried Sassoon – one of the war's earliest volunteers – wrote: 'It will be Hell to be in it, and Hell to be out of it.'

But although initial moods were high at the thought of doing one's duty for Britain, no one could ever imagine just how bloody and horrific this war would ever become. It is estimated that 192,000 British soldiers were taken prisoner during the First World War. Many were taken to camps across Europe. Many were still wounded or had been rounded up at makeshift hospitals where they had been recovering before being taken prisoner.

It had been over fifty years since Henry Dunant had written of the horrors he had seen at Solferino and since he had urged those in war

## THE TRAUMA OF CAPTIVITY

to see each other as '*tutti fratelli*' and formed the Red Cross. Yet, now his plans and his Utopian ideals seemed light years away. The stuff of dreams. Despite the Geneva Convention, cruelties abounded in prison camps during the First World War. Men were starved, beaten, forced to work in labour camps and humiliated.

In many accounts from the time, prisoners recounted being made to share a loaf of bread with several other soldiers and that, during their time in captivity, the amounts of flour in the bread became less and less until the bread was often inedible. Some soldiers were inventive at finding protein, cooking rats and mice, boiling up snails and spreading them on bread as a paste for protein.

Other soldiers who had been wounded found that their care varied from camp to camp and from soldier to soldier. Instead of beds, many wounded soldiers found themselves convalescing on straw palliasses and often bandages were torn from other soldiers' wounds and simply reused without thought to hygiene or the spread of disease.

Many returned home not only shell-shocked from conflict, but also with post-traumatic stress from their time in captivity. For others who did not receive ill treatment, the ennui was enough. One such example was a postcard sent in 1918 from Private W. Hall, who, during his civilian life, had been a member of a Mrs Hayman's Bible class in Bournemouth. From his incarceration in Germany he wrote:

> Dear Mrs Hayman, It is with the greatest of pleasure I now take in writing and hoping that this will find you and all your household in the best of health also fine weather. I must say that I am still in perfect health, weather here mild but unsettled. I should like to know if you could forward me some more books as we are getting some very long nights now and have nothing now to read. Thanking you for my parcels, Yours sincerely, Pte W. Hall.[1]

# THE FIRST WORLD WAR: 'WHILE OF UNSOUND MIND...'

Some soldiers were able to keep diaries of their time incarcerated during the First World War. One such soldier was Private David Parker, who happened to be my great-grandfather. His diaries were written in a perfectly cursive handwriting in ink. Even during his most upsetting memories, his handwriting never faltered. As mentioned in the introduction to this book, he was taken prisoner after he was bayonetted through the head at close quarters during combat. First he was taken to a nunnery in Belgium where nurses and nuns cared for him, giving him a statue of a soldier holding a flag that said *Belegt,* meaning 'occupied'. German soldiers then captured the soldiers in the nunnery-hospital and the wounded were taken prisoner.

## The diaries of POW Private David Parker, 1st Cheshire Regiment

The Germans used to visit the Convent each morning and take away all bread, milk, butter, beer, flour, bandages, chloroform, or anything they could put their hands on. There were five drafts of men taken to Germany then on 3 September they got me. We were clothed by the Belgian nuns as well as possible, put into wagons and taken to the railway station, where an officer told us we would have the pleasure of seeing Germany at their expense. Now is the beginning of my captivity.

On the afternoon of 3 September 1914, we were on our way to the railway station. The driver of the wagon I was in asked us if we would like a glass of beer. There were eight men in this wagon and we answered yes, So he pulled up outside an establishment and got us eight glasses of beer. When we had drank them, he came for the money. Imagine his surprise when we said we had none and told him the Germans would pay for them. He gabbled something but being unable to comprehend what it was it did not worry us at all. Then we formed up against a wall. The women of the village came and gave us all cigarettes, tobacco, chocolate, matches, eggs, handkerchiefs. But as soon as the Huns saw them they banged our heads against the wall and called us by the favourite name of English swine and took everything we had from us. We were then put in, or should I say kicked in, to the train. I got in a carriage where one man had to lie full stretch. When the German officers saw I was standing up he pleasantly said: 'Come here, Englishman, get into one of the other carriages where you can sit down comfortably.'

I was going to obey when his mind must have taken another turn and he kicked me out of that one and followed me and kicked me into another. I got in and burst out laughing. The officer jumped in after me, pulled out his revolver and clapped it against my head. If he had pulled the trigger I should have had to laugh, but he contented himself by smacking me across the face and bawling: 'Swine, swine!'

It was the impression of the Germans at that time that Englishmen were a lot of cut-throats. They accused of us taking the eyes out of the German wounded with the marker spike of our jack knife. I discovered the carriage I was in was next to a carriage full of German wounded sent from their firing line. We had six men and two German sentries in each carriage and away we went bound for that living hell called Sennelager.

It was a long railway journey. We started at 3 pm on the 3rd and arrived at Sennelager at 10 pm the night of the 5th. The train would occasionally stop so that the sentry could get sandwiches and coffee but they never gave us any. I have not yet met or saw a good German. The first I do, I will shoot him before he goes bad. I poked my head out of the carriage window and had my coat and cap off at the time and the women on the platform who were giving cigars to the sentries must have mistaken me for a German because she handed me a box of cigars which I eagerly snatched. Then the train began to move out of the station, just as they discovered I was one of their pet swines. But it was too late. I emptied out the cigars and flung her the empty box, then set about distributing cigars to the boys in the carriage.

## THE FIRST WORLD WAR: 'WHILE OF UNSOUND MIND...'

We pulled up at Cologne where they gave us all a small basin of hot water, or what was termed soup, and a half loaf of the blackest and sourest bread I have ever tasted. This was the first bite of food for 52 hours and although I was very hungry the majority of the men could not eat the sour bread and it was flung through the window. Our next stop was Munster, there the Germans received food and drink. There were two sisters of mercy on the platform giving out hot coffee to the sentries. They motioned to me to come down and get a cup, which I did, one of them handed me the cup and just as I was about to take it from her, she suddenly found out that I was English. She let out an unearthly yell of 'Swine!' and spat straight into my face. I closed my fist. I was about to strike her when up came a Red Cross orderly with a revolver in each hand, but with a running kick in my rear he lifted me back to my carriage. When we arrived at Senne, all the town was lit up, flags and banners flying and great rejoicing. One would think they had captured the whole of the British forces instead of a few disabled men, and they were taken from hospital. We were marched to a great open space or compound amid the taunts and jeers of the German civilians. There were some of the Gordon Highlanders with us and one could hear the Germans saying 'Fraus' thinking they were women. We were formed into two lines and searched. An English civilian was acting as interpreter and he told us if we had any knives, razors, maps, compasses of any description to hand them over or if you are found with anything on you after being searched you will be shot. Then there was a titter, for someone said: 'What, again?' My razor was concealed down my puttee so I took it out and hit the blade against a waggon wheel then handed it over as useless to me or them. We were then told we could lie down in the sand and go to sleep until morning and that there were sentries posted every six feet around the camp and any man found walking about would be shot. We asked if we could get something to eat but were told it was too late but we could get a good breakfast next morning. So we had to grin and bear it. Next morning, 7 September, we were again inspected by a German officer that could speak English. He asked me one of the silliest questions I ever heard. 'Why did you come out to fight your cousins the Germans?' Which I readily answered: 'Because I was made in England.' For that I received a well-planted smack across the mouth.

The men asked him what time we would get breakfast and he said arrangements were being made to give us hot soup about 12 o'clock so we had to be content until midday. We received a small bowl of soup, a slice of bread and a small piece of their famous German sausage. At 6 pm we got coffee, or rather burnt barley without sugar or milk, and another piece of bread. We were afterwards formed up to get straw to sleep on as each man passed the officer gave him about as much straw as he could fit in his cap. We again slept in the open. Through the night it rained heavy so it was a matter of sitting up back to back. With sitting in the soft sand, we were making small hollows which would fill up with water and the seat of our trousers – those that had trousers – would get uncomfortably wet. Although it was unpleasant, some would sing, some would tell yarns, others would come out with witty sayings such as 'roll on furlough', 'sit still and you won't get half as wet' or 'if the sentries can stick it, we can'. My mate and I had one overcoat between us which we covered ourselves with and fell asleep. But during the night, somebody that was short of covering kindly lifted ours away.

Next morning we were taken for a bath at 5 am. About twenty men would go at a time, strip off, put the clothing (with strict orders not to put in any article made of leather) into a fumigator, then parade in front of the doctor, be inspected, then take a bath which lasted ten minutes. Afterwards, standing in a cold wet room one and a half hours waiting for our clothing which would come back damp with steam. French and English were together. While I was dressing, I missed my boots and found that some affectionate froggy had placed his boots into the fumigator. The result was they had shrunk and shrivelled up to a quarter of their size so he kindly took mine and left me his.

## THE FIRST WORLD WAR: 'WHILE OF UNSOUND MIND...'

I reported my loss to a German but neither of us could find them. So I got a pair of rubber slippers from a corporal in my regiment. That is only one incident of the crafty froggy. We then went and had all our hair, beards and moustaches cut completely off which made us look more like prisoners. On the way back from the bath, I saw for the first time the German method of punishment. An English civilian negro was tied to a tree by the ankles, wrists and neck, bare-headed. He was left in that position in the glare of a blazing sun for six hours. As we were passing him he called out to us: 'Stick it, soldiers. We are all British.'

At one o'clock we got soup and bread but the men had begun to distrust the Germans and although very hungry there were rumours of poison being placed in the water and soup and many left it untouched. After dinner we were told to fall in for work. At first the men fought shy of such an idea as working for the Germans but when we saw the numbers of armed sentries we could hardly help ourselves. Then we got the command to fall in by our own sergeant major and 500 of us were taken to work in a field about 6km from the camp with two sentries to each four men. We commenced to cut down trees, and dig all the roots. Then commenced the longest, hardest, filthiest, most indescribable five months I ever experienced.

We had to parade every morning at 5 am no matter what the weather was like, then off to work and return at 6 pm without a morsel of food until we came back to camp. Then we would receive a small loaf between six men and a basin of soup each. The bad weather had begun and there was rain every day. I was still wearing my rubber slippers, sleeping at night on filthy wet straw, creeping and bleeding with scratching at the lice on my clothing and body. No brushes, no soap, no razor, only one shirt, no socks, but small pieces of cloth for toe rags, nothing but work on an empty stomach until on the 2 November I was taken to hospital with rheumatics in the legs, where I remained on my bed for six weeks. The doctor visited us every morning but they had nothing to give us in regards to treatment. We were told to lie in bed and keep warm which could easily be done by all the rubbing and scratching our verminous bodies. There were terrible sufferings. Men of all nationalities were being carried into hospital every hour of the day with rheumatism, colic, cramp, fever. Our doctors reported four cases of death through starvation. It was a common sight to see men stealing a cap full of potato peelings and cooking them or what we termed 'drumming up' in a stove made of an old biscuit tin. I came out of hospital back to the camp where a few huts had been erected and where we were issued with a straw mattress to be placed on the floor. The bread ration had by now gone to four men per loaf but only for a fortnight. It then went up again to six men per loaf for a month then to ten to a loaf made by a far worse quality of flour, rye, potatoes and heather. We were on a starvation diet. There were no sanitary arrangements. Our lavatory consisted of a small trench dug just outside the huts and every Sunday civilians came up to see the Englanders – officers' wives and so-called women taking photos and snapshots of our men at the latrines and urinals and they boasted of culture.

About January the parcels of foodstuffs began to arrive in small numbers. At first, one would see about 300 men clamouring round a small piece of paper with about four names for parcels but more and more came each week until in about two months' time they were issuing 2,000 parcels a day. What a Godsend a parcel of food and clothing was. We had foot to eat, although bread and cakes were sometimes green and mouldy, they were eaten just the same. Not a scrap was wasted. We had soap to wash ourselves – a great luxury. Shirts, vests, drawers, socks, scarves, gloves to change with and discard our old rags. By now the Germans had begun to look upon us in a different light as something human instead of savages. So they sent large batches of sentries to the front and other camps until we were left with one sentry to each six men. We left the huts and were put into stables with a cold cement floor and iron manger. We were there a week when a man belonging to another stable stole a loaf and ran through the stable I belonged to.

## THE FIRST WORLD WAR: 'WHILE OF UNSOUND MIND...'

The sentry fired at him and missed so the Sergeant Major said if we did not tell who the man was, he would punish all in the stable. Nobody spoke, so he took us and gave us two hours running around the compound without a halt. A Sergeant Major of the Suffolk Regiment led the way and took it very easy. We had run for one and a half hours when the commander of the camp came on the scene. He asked had we had any dinner. When he was told no, he said we must be dismissed. They opened the gate of the compound. The Sergeant Major shouted: 'Step out!' and away we chased as fast as our legs would carry us. The commandant was heard to say that it's useless trying to punish an Englishman with physical exercise because they like it.

Then came a time when if a man did any wrong he was tied to the post for two hours and would receive no soup but would get two rations of bread. So one day when I was terribly hungry I went and tied myself to the post for two hours, got two rations of bread and my soup when I went up to the stable. But that game got played out and there were too many of us doing it. But we had come down to a state where we feared nothing and respected nothing. Men had to keep side stepping to keep their bellies balanced. The spirit of the troops was marvellous. They kept up their hearts as only Britishers know how. On 21 January '15, I was again carried to hospital with rheumatic fever where I remained for a month. I came out of hospital on 23 February and went back to slavery helping to make another camp known as Stone Muchel, better known as Siberia. This work continued every day up to me leaving Senne.

On 1 July 1915, a couple of days before leaving Senne, I and two more men went into a field to steal some carrots when a sentry fired at us, missed and hit a Frenchman about 200 yards on our right killing him. We got a chocking off for it, but as they spoke German and us not understanding the language, it made little impression. On the morning of 1 July 1915 we said goodbye to Senne for Dülmen.

We arrived safe and sound after seeing the sights of the surrounding country passing hundreds of wheat fields all fallen down and useless with the heavy rains. We got to Dülmen which reminded one of a large bird cage with its 8ft high barbed wire all around the camp. Once in we were doomed to hard work. We commenced next day, shovelling sand and making the hills and hollows all level which lasted about three months. Then we had to set to to make another camp. I got a job as a joiner helping to rig up the huts and many a happy hour I spent knocking in about twelve nails where two should go, and two where twelve should go, burying packets of nails, hammers, saws, wood chisels and all kinds of tools, writing inscriptions on the lathes of the huts such as 'These huts were built by St George's Men – hoping they fall on the first German that occupies them.'

This work lasted for seven months. There were at first 600 men passing through the gate for work – English and French – and in about a month the Germans had their work cut out trying to get twenty of our men to go to work. The sentries were the prisoners and we had the upper hand. We could do almost as we liked. If a sentry bullied us, we would report him to the commandant and he would send him to the front. I remained at Dülmen until 10 April.

I commenced work at a brewer on the 11th but that wouldn't suit. I refused to work. So I was sent to a farm from 12 April to 16 June. I worked on other farms, messed about doing more damage than I was worth until 31 July, I reported sick with my ear and I was sent to Minden and admitted into hospital where I stayed until 7 October. I came out of hospital on the 7th and put on the list to see the Swiss Commission and given a ticket for no work. Next morning I was warned to get ready to proceed to Friedrichsfeld Convalescent Camp. We left Minden at 7.15 am and arrived at our destination at 9 pm, Our party consisted of mainly badly wounded men, fingers off, legs twisted and short, pieces blown out of their shoulders and various other injuries. We were marched through a network of lanes and arrived at the Stone Quarries. Next morning every man agreed not to work until we had seen a doctor. We turned out at 6 am. We were given a bowl of cold barley which no pig could eat, then we got

## THE FIRST WORLD WAR: 'WHILE OF UNSOUND MIND...'

orders to fall in for work but the cry went up: 'Be British! And no man would move.

So they placed us all in a small compound and left us until midday then we were taken to see a German doctor. Of our twenty-eight men, seven were sent straight away as unfit for work. The others, he said, were fit and must work. They took us down to the quarries. I said: Every man must do his own, I am going to do mine and that is not to work. Not even if they killed me.

I got as far as the workings, and saw waggons marked Krupp and Co. That did it. I sat down holding my head. The sentry came and told me to 'arbeit'. I said I did not understand. He showed me how to pick and fill the waggons. I said I was sick and not strong enough to work. So he took me back to the under officers. He let me go to bed for the afternoon. Next morning I went and saw the doctor again and of course I must work. I came back and got into bed again. Two sentries dragged me out and I was placed two paces from the wall with my hands behind me. They told me to bend in a stooping position until my nose was about half an inch from a window sill, there to remain for four hours. Every now and then the under officer would walk past me giving my head a little knock sending my nose onto the window sill. I would not work in the afternoon so I got the same punishment as the morning. I was left without food. Next morning again I reported sick but again received the same treatment and was told I must work. While going across a locomotive track, I fainted but was restored quickly by a brutal kick full in the face. I went down to the workings just to show willing and lifted about twenty stones into the waggon, but it was useless. I couldn't do any more. I hung out until the men had finished at 7 pm then walked to the under officer and told him I was too sick to work. He said he had orders that if any man refused to work he could shoot him without trial. With that a sentry began to bully me. He fixed his bayonet on his rifle. I threw open my jacket, bared my chest and shoved myself against it and told him to stick it through. That frightened the sentry and I then asked the under officer to carry on with his shooting as I would be far better off. I would have plenty of sleep and no work. I got a few kicks and punches. I then went to my bed and remained there for seven days and nights without a morsel of food, not even a drink of water. On the eighth day the doctor came to me and said I must go to the Lazarette and a French man gave me two biscuits and a drink of chocolate. Then on 17 November I was passed by two German doctors and a Swiss medical officer fit to proceed to Switzerland. I stayed in the camp a fortnight then was sent to Constance, remaining there for ten days. The medical board were not ready for us so we were packed off down the line to a place called Rastatt and placed in a fortress among about 3,000 French civilians – men, women and children. After being there sixteen days we were sent back to Constance. We had not the slightest idea of getting to Switzerland then. We stayed in the carriages a little while, got a little to eat and then were transferred to another train where the Swiss officials took us over into their charge. Two minutes afterwards I was crossing the frontier. We all shook hands with ourselves. My feelings of having my fetters cut from me are indescribable. It was like being in another world. We had a grand reception at Zurich and also at Berne, arriving In Murren on the 14 December 1916.

When Private David Parker returned to Britain, he resettled in Stockport, Lancashire, with his wife and two children. He died in his sixties. Little is known of how he settled back into civilian life and whether his time as a prisoner of war haunted him. From most accounts he was a decent, quiet man who was never out of work. There was no talk of violence or alcohol abuse. Like so many ex-prisoners of war of the time, it appears he kept his feelings to himself, except for in his diary.

In comparison to many other soldiers of the Great War who were taken prisoner, Private Parker was one of the fortunate ones. He settled, had a family, returned to work. If he had demons or flashbacks or post-traumatic stress, he didn't show it. Yet many soldiers returned unable to escape the horror they had endured. Some

## THE FIRST WORLD WAR: 'WHILE OF UNSOUND MIND...'

were unable to work. Others unable to find suitable lodgings. Some were still suffering from 'nerves' or 'headaches' which would later be described as shell-shock. Newspapers of the time detailed the many tragic ends of men who simply were unable to come to terms with, to talk about, or to express what they had endured as prisoners of war:

> Suicide of returned prisoner of war: Badly Treated in Germany. At Paddington Mr Oswald held an inquest on Charles Summerfield (25), French polisher, of Grove Road, Holloway. His brother, an instrument maker, of Avenue, Hendon, said the deceased was badly treated when a prisoner of war in Germany and starved that when released he had the appearance of a skeleton. Lately he was out of work and was distressed over a girl to whom he was engaged. Monday visited witness at Hendon and soon after he was found groaning and sent him to the hospital suffering from an irritant poison. He died next day, and afterwards a packet of bichromate of potash was found in his pocket. Florence Ithell, of Gloucester Street Clerkenwell, leather stitcher, said she had been engaged to deceased for twelve months. Lately he had been shaky and nervous. They had no trouble and were happy. The night he took poison was very strange, and ran away from her without wishing her Goodbye. Dr Day, of St Mary's Hospital, said that death was due to poisoning bichromate of potassium. The Coroner said there was no reflection be cast on the girl, and recorded verdict of suicide while of unsound mind.[2]

Elsewhere ex-soldiers who had been held prisoner in Europe were finding ways to end their own suffering:

> A prisoner of war hanging in a barn: Nutley farmer's sad end.

# THE TRAUMA OF CAPTIVITY

> The village of Nutley was disturbed on Friday when it became known that Mr John Henry Darnet a well known farmer of Nutley Inn Farm had been found hanging in a barn. Deceased, who was about 35 years of age, was a prisoner during the Great War. He subsequently met with a serious motor incident.... Deceased was a prisoner in Germany from 1914 to 1919 who since then had behaved strangely at times and complained of his head. He was a man of strange moods and would sometimes say strange things to them but had never threatened to take his life and was very 'down' on that sort of thing. His mental condition would be accounted for partly, no doubt, from being interned all that time and he may have had shell-shock and also concussion. All these things would have caused injury to the brain. The coroner returned a verdict of suicide while of unsound mind.[3]

Of course, among the reports of suffering and ill mental health, there were the tales of stiff upper lip, of soldiers coming home and resuming their studies, going straight back into work, having relationships or ending relationships. In one court hearing of maintenance from a husband to his estranged wife, he said: 'I was a prisoner of war for eleven months and had a better time then than I have had with her during the last three months.'[4]

This light-hearted quip at this husband's maintenance hearing would have brought about a smile under many a moustache. But beneath those smiles, men who had been a prisoner knew too well that this was not the consensus. Many of those who had not suffered cruelty had been starved or overworked instead, often returning emaciated or with long-lasting health damage. But more often it was the unseen damage that caused problems for returning men. Some prisoners, as one newspaper article details, had even turned against their own during captivity:

## THE FIRST WORLD WAR: 'WHILE OF UNSOUND MIND...'

> Cruelty charges: Remarkable evidence was given at Woolwich yesterday at the resume court martial of Private H. Owen of the Middlesex Regiment attached to the 4th Reserve Brigade, RFA Owen was charged with 'disgraceful conduct of a cruel kind' in that at a prisoner of war camp at Marets, while acting as interpreter, he was party to his fellow prisoners of war being deprived of their rations. He was also charged with standing by while his fellow prisoners were whipped, after they had complained to him that they were ill; and also with himself striking some of his fellow prisoners.

The article continues in great detail of the cruelty Private Owen inflicted upon his fellow prisoners, including stripping and beating them, hitting them with rifle butts and depriving them of rations for twelve hours after being forced to work.

> Witness for the defence said that his opinion was that Owen caused the British prisoners to suffer in order that he might curry favour with the Germans.
> 'The Commandant of the camp, who could speak English,' added the witness, 'told us: "You are in hell now. I am the devil and I will provide the fire. Owen is your master and if you do not obey him you will be severely punished.[5]

Whether Owens behaved this way to his fellow inmates out of cruelty or to curry favour, it demonstrates the strata of hierarchy in the prison camps even between men of the same rank and on the same side. This sense of not knowing who one could trust must have made the whole situation even more unbearable.

And yet, at a psychiatric conference called the War Neurology Congress held in Munich in 1916, psychiatrists decided that captivity during war 'protected' against mental illness, rather than invoked it. Their belief was that, away from enemy lines, away from the fear and noise and horror of battle, captive prisoners of war were unlikely to suffer from 'shell-shock' or any other kind of neurosis and were more protected than the average soldier. But Germany had captured far more prisoners that Britain or France and by 1915, over one million prisoners were being held there. There was simply not enough space for all these men at first and so many were housed in other locations, or even slept rough in fields until camps were built. Men were also used in mining, agricultural work and other manual labour roles and many were forced to work near the shelling by the front lines. So it is not true that these men were wholly 'protected' from the war by being prisoners.

Back in Britain, returning prisoners of war were not helped by the fact that many of them returned to even worse poverty than they had left behind. The average foot soldier who enlisted would have been working class and of low rank. Immediately after the First World War, Britain, along with the United States, fell into recession, complicated further by all the returning military men who now needed jobs. Factories that had been utilised to make wartime goods now had to close and re-tool back to pre-war enterprises. When these men returned, those who could found work but for others, whose minds perhaps still rang out with the booms of bombs, or whose hands shook with the jitters of spending every night in a freezing, damp trench, it was not so easy.

> Family of seven in mud hut: Plight of man who was prisoner of war.
>
> The pitiable condition of an ex-serviceman, his wife and their five children who were discovered living in a mud hut at Bromley Woods, Catford, was related at Greenwich. Before Mr Gattie were James William Baulch and his wife Harriet who were charged with

exposing their children in a manner likely to injure their health. A constable described how he found the whole family asleep in the hut, which was built of turf, plastered with mud and roofed with corrugated iron. The rain was coming through the roof. Baulch said: 'I was turned out of my rooms on account of the children. I went to the Lambeth Guardians but they would not take the children without my wife and myself. I am able-bodied and my wife does a bit of housework. I am doing the best I can for them. I served in the war and was a prisoner of war in Germany for four years and this is what I get.'[6]

Men returning from war who had been declared unfit due to, or aggravated by, military service could apply for a disability pension. There were six pension classes based on rank ranging from class 1 for a warrant officer down to troopers, privates and gunners. The amount awarded was increased if the soldier had children and a wife and if on returning from war he was earning less than he had earned pre-war, a top-up was sometimes granted. But the conditions listed in the acceptable disabilities include conditions such as heart dilation, loss of limbs, mobility issues and so on. Mental health was not a 'disability' to be considered. Some men tried to forget what they had been through. Others had to face it once more. One moving account of how a prisoner was able to revisit the place he was held captive just four years after the war ended in 1923 was written by Daniel Griffiths in the *Manchester Evening News*. His colleague invited him to Germany to attend the races and Griffiths later wrote in the newspaper:

Ghosts of Ruhleben: a prisoner of war revisits the scene of his captivity:
In the centre was the usual expanse of grass with a small pond. It still showed patches of wear ('that's where

the goal posts were,' said my friend), at the far end some cabbage patches ('I planted one of these,' he explained) and on the far side the third class stand and enclosure. 'That's where they dumped all the rubbish, sorted the old paper and collected all the string,' he explained. 'But I've never been as far as that.'... 'My word,' he said. 'This place is full of ghosts.'

He began to tell me something of the strange life that the prisoners led. Brought from all over Germany at the outset of war, drawn from all classes, and inspired by the wildest divergence of feelings, they had settled down to life in the closest intimacy in Ruhleben. Four to a room was the rule. The course and its buildings had soon become more than a town – it was a universe. There was no outside for the prisoner. The world for him was bounded on the north, south, east and west by barbed wire. The fields in the distance were as far off as the planet Mars. One of the prisoners had a telescope and he used to let his fellow prisoners look through it at two pence a time. My friend showed me windows in the back of the grandstand; the men used to climb onto one another's backs to see a little farther. 'Once in 1916,' he remarked, 'I saw a girl through there and waved to her and she waved back.'

That was the grim side of the story, to be placed beside those days when the parcels did not turn up because the ship bringing them had been submarined and the camp was reduced to living on ship's biscuits or the trials of prisoners for some petty delinquency before the camp had achieved self-government, or the suicides. 'When a man gazes on the same scene day after day, year after year,' said my friend, 'it begins to hurt your eyes. We couldn't all remain quite sane. Some just gave it up.'[7]

## THE FIRST WORLD WAR: 'WHILE OF UNSOUND MIND...'

Returning to the scene where one was kept prisoner might well have been a tonic and helpful for a man's mental health. Yet for those who did not have the means to travel back to Europe and face their demons, their preoccupation was simply surviving in the here and now. Many prisoners of war returned to nothing – no home, no job, no income and a shattered economy as well as a housing crisis.

> Ex-soldier living in cowshed at Atherstone. At a meeting of the Atherstone Rural Council, reference was made to the acute housing shortage. The straits to which are reduced are illustrated above. An ex-soldier who was a prisoner of war for 18 months in Germany is living with his wife and two children in a cowshed. The living quarters being so small, part of the furniture has to be stored under cover outside.[8]

This account was written in 1923, more than four years after the war had ended. These men, who had endured suffering no one around them could comprehend, were often reduced to living in this way – in sheds, in outhouses, in rooms or in squalor – dealing with not only finding enough money to buy food to eat, but also while dealing with their own declining mental health.

However, in the years after their return from being prisoners in the Great War those men who had the means often revisited the places they had been held captive. Was this cathartic? A form of exposure to overcome the nightmares?

> Burnley businessman revisits German village: After a lapse of ten years, a Burnley business man Mr Smith Heap, who is chairman of the 2/2 East Lancashire Field Ambulance Old Boys' Association Committee recently revisited Oberkirn, a village in the German province of Hunsruck, Rhineland where he was a prisoner during

> the war, and worked on a farm with a number of English and Russian soldiers. During his holiday he worked on the farm where he used to work as a prisoner of war and assisted in the hayfield the farmer who was himself a prisoner of war in this country during the war.⁹

Perhaps revisiting the place they were held captive was a step forward to coming to terms with their incarceration.

Class and wealth, it seemed, as in so many other areas of society, meant that some ex-prisoners of war would be doomed to suffer more than those who had more means than them. This class divide meant that the working class, lowest-ranking soldiers were often the ones neglected and had their mental health needs ignored. But another consideration aside from the mental scarring, was the poor physical health of prisoners of war when they came home. Often wounds received on the battlefield were not treated properly if a soldier was taken prisoner. If this didn't kill a man in the camp itself, it led to lasting effects – often for life.

> A man who was a prisoner of war in Germany died recently and left four children. Owing to the fact that the man was a prisoner for four and a half years he said it was difficult to get any information for pension purposes. The man was captured by the Germans at the first battle of Mons and he was then taken into Germany. He was brutally ill-treated and struck by a German sentry and his jaw broken and he was fixed up with lead teeth. All the time he was a prisoner the food and conditions were absolutely wretched and now the man had broken down and died of cancer. It was practically impossible to get any record of the man while he was a prisoner of war in Germany. He was discharged in 1920.¹⁰

## THE FIRST WORLD WAR: 'WHILE OF UNSOUND MIND...'

For the many who had already been of ill health before enlisting in the army, their chances of living a long life on their return were even slimmer.

> We regret to record the death of Mr Thomas Gilliat, a young Spilsby tradesman ... and his demise at the early age of 25 years is much regretted in East Lincolnshire where he had made many friends. Deceased had been in poor health for some time but the end came suddenly. He was a promising and enterprising tradesman and had an excellent war record. He early answered the call of King and country and did service with a Yorkshire regiment 'over there'. It was while acting as a signaller and upon an arduous and perilous duty that he was captured by the Boche, most of his comrades either being slain or captured in this particular action. For many months he remained a prisoner of war and the experiences he underwent no doubt undermined his constitution. At the time of his capture by the enemy, he was severely wounded and could barely be prevailed upon to chat about his experiences as a prisoner of war, preferring rather to make that unhappy chapter of his life a sealed book, we gather that his wounds received little or no attention.[11]

With no NHS – this did not start until 1948 – these men would have had to pay to see a doctor about any conditions which might have arisen from being a prisoner of war. Without the means to even secure lodgings, these men did not have the money for a doctor's appointment to discuss festering wounds or stomach complaints after being held prisoner in dire conditions. Another post-war consideration for returning POWs was simply the lack of employment. At the start of the war, many men had left apprenticeships, new jobs or first positions in their chosen career and had returned to find those jobs filled or gone. Even as women returned to their position in the home and men took their places again as breadwinner, jobs could not always be found. Ex-soldier Joseph John Keen was 35 when he committed suicide when his job working in a bootmaker's shop was not kept open for him on his return. The local and national papers of the 1920s were littered with suicides of ex-prisoners of war. One such story was of Edward Matthews, a private in the East Lancashire Regiment who was out of work on his return from captivity due to neurasthenia, an out-dated term used in the post First World War era to describe any condition characterised by fatigue, headaches, irritability or emotional disturbance. Matthews had been taken prisoner at Mons and was held captive for four years. He then shot himself back home in Shepherd's Bush after the war after being 'so poorly fed [in captivity] that but for parcels received from home he would have starved.'[12]

Of the Matthews case, the coroner said of the parcels he had received during captivity: 'He was lucky to get them. Many were stolen. Among civilised nations it was customary to feed their prisoners of war but of course the Germans never thought of such a thing.'

In a letter, Matthews wrote: 'I knew this would be my end.' On a pension form he scribbled: 'The Germans wanted to know why the English treated their prisoners so well and I simply answered: "Christian charity. Good old England."' A verdict of suicide while of unsound mind was returned.[13]

Suicide 'while of unsound mind' is a phrase that littered newspaper reports on inquests into men's deaths. Often it was only during the inquest that those around the deceased had any idea what he had been going through since their incarceration. For men who had endured the war and been imprisoned, the return home had been their only dream. When that return was not how they had imagined it, they often could just not cope anymore. One Hampshire-based ex-soldier and prisoner took his life in 1920, two years after the end of the war:

## THE FIRST WORLD WAR: 'WHILE OF UNSOUND MIND...'

> The deceased was a discharged soldier who lived with his mother and step-father. James McKay, the stepfather, said that his stepson joined the Rifle Brigade in 1890, served in the African War, and was afterwards discharged. In 1914, however, he again joined the service and was wounded three times in France besides being interned for eighteen months as a prisoner of war in Germany. Upon his return to England, he joined the Royal Engineers in July 1919 and served until May 1920 when he was discharged as medically unfit.[14]

The ex-prisoner of war had told his mother and stepfather he was going to Winchester to try and join the army again. A carter had been travelling along the road when he'd found the serviceman's body in a copse. A post-mortem found he had taken cyanide. A verdict of suicide was given again – 'while of unsound mind'.

The phrase litters the suicide verdicts in coroners' courts throughout the newspapers in the 1920s. Soldiers who had experienced cruelty, torture, starvation and captivity were simply not given the tools to cope when they returned home. And even those who could return to a job or similar position to the one they held before the war, were often hiding their true feelings of how they were coping. One such example was that of Lance Corporal G. Wingate who had been a prisoner of war and his rather matter-of-fact letter:

> 'Dear old Joe – I am fed up with life in general. I am off. Give my apologies to the boys. Best regards to yourself.'
>
> This was the letter left by Lance Corporal G Wingate, Military Police, stationed at Dover, who shot himself on Saturday with a revolver. At the inquest yesterday it was stated that his conduct was satisfactory, and he had nothing to worry about, but was disappointed regarding

a training course. A verdict of suicide while of unsound mind was returned.

A similar finding has come to in the case of Lance Sergeant Henry John Palmer (36), 2nd Battalion, Green Howards also stationed at Dover who had been a prisoner of war in Germany for four years and who also shot himself on Saturday with a rifle just before going out on parade. At the inquest it was stated that he had expressed the belief that he was slowly being poisoned.[15]

In 1929, eleven years after the end of the First World War, the second Geneva Convention was drawn up replacing the Hague Convention of 1907. Further provisions for war at sea were now included, which involved also protecting hospital ships from being mined and shelled. Articles five and six of the 1929 convention importantly stress the treatment of prisoners on capture. It stated that if prisoners were too ill to comply, all they must give were their names and rank but not be forced to give any more information. Later articles stated that food must be of a similar quality and quantity to that of the 'belligerent's own soldiers' and that prisoners must not be denied food as punishment.[16]

Those who signed – forty-seven countries, including Germany – stated that each prisoner would be fed adequately, treated humanely and had the right to correspondence and parcels.

Seeing it written down and printed in such a clear way seemed to make a mockery of all that had come before. Why weren't prisoners given the right to be fed adequately during the First World War? What had changed since that first signing of the Geneva Convention? How had war changed what governments could agree to in peacetime – basic things such as human rights, dignity and access to food and water?

After the horrors of the Great War, the world was hopeful for change.

# Chapter Three

# Psychological Intervention

'I was doomed to spend the rest of my life paying the bill for all those shells and tanks and bullets and the state of mind used to provide an armour.'

Wilfred Bion, psychoanalyst

'John McMahon, the Harthill miner who went missing on his way to work on 9 August, and who suffered from loss of memory, has been found drowned in an old quarry at Whitburn. He suffered from shell-shock and was a prisoner of war in Germany. His wife's death two months ago left him greatly depressed. There are four children.'

*Edinburgh Evening News* – Saturday, 21 August 1920

The initial repatriation of First World War prisoners meant many returning soldiers were still, at first, on a high. The Red Cross had been negotiating the repatriation of prisoners of war abroad since the end of 1914, with the severely wounded being the first priority. The Red Cross appealed to the belligerents: 'All nations have equal interest to see their own come back in sound health in both body and mind. Our conscience rises strongly against the extension of a detention that could deprive Europe of millions of human beings.'[1]

The ICRC worked tirelessly to appeal for prisoners to be given back or exchanged. From Britain and the Commonwealth it was estimated that 192,000 prisoners of war had been taken. Ahead of its time, the Red Cross had appealed to belligerents in 1916 that even those of poor mental state also be considered for early release, as well as those with physical complaints. Gradually, as the war ended, British prisoners of war were repatriated via neutral Switzerland. The initial focus was simply on getting these men home, but many of them had seen and experienced horrors that would emerge later, after the initial elation of being freed had ebbed away.

After the First World War many ex-prisoners of war felt they had fallen into a chasm but so many were unable to find the words. Back at home, some were unable to find work, unable to secure proper lodgings, and some unable to forge relationships. Although, strangely, the suicide rate had dropped during and just after the First World War – something experts attributed to men feeling more socially integrated and 'useful' during a war and a sense of national cohesion – the post-traumatic stress was something many men felt they had to live with and endure at a time where men did not discuss emotions.

But one man – himself also a soldier in the First World War – was to forge change. Wilfred Bion was still a teenager when he had fought in the war in Northern France. He had served as a tank commander and his bravery had won him the Legion of Honour. But he would later explain how his experiences on the battlefield haunted him.

After returning from war, Bion studied medicine at University College London where he developed a growing interest in psychoanalysis. While waiting to start his degree, Bion wrote his memoirs entitled *Diary, France*. The book, a harrowing read, documents his time as a tank commander between 1917 and 1918, which he dedicated to his parents in lieu of 'letters I should have written'. His diaries cover the attack at Ypres in 1917 when his tank became bogged down in mud. In the hot, cramped interior of the tank, Bion was a sitting duck, hearing the bombs drop around him and the whistle of bullets all around.

In another excerpt, he recalls the Battle of Cambrai, during which 44,000 men were killed, and how one of his troop's tanks burst into flames, killing the entire crew. He wrote: 'I got out of the tank and rather dreamily watched the crew rolling about inside – some coughing, some groaning and one man lying almost still enough to be dead....' Although the memoir is written in a very straight, matter-of-fact, unemotional tone, Bion's experiences of war, he would later write, traumatised him and haunted him. But those same experiences would later help him forge a distinguished career as one of the most respected psychoanalysts in history as well as helping many traumatised ex-prisoners of the Second World War, as we shall see later in this book.

The young Bion studied under surgeon and neurosurgeon Wilfred Trotter in London, who had a great impact on his later work on group psychology. Trotter, who arguably coined the term 'herd instinct', was author of the great work *Instinct of the Herd in Peace and War 1916–1919*, which features a collection of essays written over fourteen years. His theory was, simply, that man has a herd instinct and will always inevitably favour the group or herd over the will of the individual. This in particular explained how so many men could 'join up' for war, risk their lives for war and put the group – the Army – ahead of their own needs and survival. Trotter was, first and foremost, a surgeon and debuted a theory about post-traumatic amnesia after a concussion. His work was important because after the First World War many soldiers and ex-POWs suffered what was termed at the time 'neurasthenia' – basically anxiety, neurosis, a state of fear and headaches. Trotter's theories said that blunt traumatic injury to the brain could cause these effects, particularly in soldiers after battle. Therefore many soldiers and ex-prisoners who suffered headaches and anxiety were turned away from receiving help because they might not have realised they also had a genuine physical reason – concussion – for their symptoms. This only compounded the issue for many ex-prisoners of war who felt there was no one to turn to for both their physical and mental needs. Would anyone even believe them?

Indeed, many working-class soldiers who displayed signs of neurasthenia, or anxiety, or 'shell-shock' were simply deposited in what were called at the time 'pauper lunatic asylums'. Asylums at the time were divided into pauper asylums and non-pauper asylums. The poor were of course sent to pauper lunatic asylums where some often died within months.

In one asylum in Cane Hill, Croydon, forty soldiers suffering from psychiatric disturbances were deposited and when they died were buried in a nearby cemetery without military fanfare.[2]

When the First World War began there were over 100,000 people certified as pauper lunatics[3] and there were 102 registered lunatic asylums. When injured soldiers and ex-POWs began returning from the Front as the war dragged on, that number increased. Many working-class soldiers had no help, no financial support, no job or home in place and were lumped in with 'pauper lunatics' and placed in asylums. However, the public attitude towards serving soldiers and particularly prisoners of war, was that if they were placed in lunatic asylums they should at least be differentiated from civilian 'mad men'. So in many hospitals and asylums, returning soldiers and ex-POWs were given special uniforms to distinguish them from other inmates. Yet, as the war continued and more and more men returned not of sound mind, the inmates numbers swelled. Worryingly, under the 1890 Lunacy Act – which continued until 1959 – a 'lunatic' could be sent to an asylum on the authority of just one person.[4] This meant that many soldiers and returning POWs were committed to lunatic asylums for displaying anxiety, nerves, shell-shock, inability to sleep or because of turning to drink or violence, often on the word of one individual. Yet, as the numbers in these institutions continued to rise, soldiers who were not as 'damaged' as others, or were quieter, or non-violent were simply released or sent to workhouses. Over in Germany, the authorities had found themselves with a much larger number of prisoners of war than they had ever planned for. As a result, conditions for prisoners in Germany during the First World War were often harsh and uncomfortable. Many prisoners slept in cold hangars or in outdoor tents. Many had to dig holes for warmth. Soon the number of soldier prisoners on German soil reached 652,000[5] and British soldiers would have had to share lodgings with soldiers from France, Russia, Canada, Belgium and other nations. By August 1916, there were 1,625,000 prisoners of war in Germany.[6]

In these camps, food was sparse. Soldiers often recalled having a meagre bread ration at the beginning or end of each day, or of sharing a loaf with several other men. As war dragged on many POWs became malnourished losing not only weight but centimetres in height and spinal damage, causing irreparable damage to their health. When they returned to Britain if they escaped being sent to a lunatic asylum, their physical health suffered instead. Some were unable to eat properly on their return, others unable to sleep, so used were they to sleeping on straw, or the floor, or covered with lice. This condition, so ubiquitous among men returning from captivity in the war, was now termed 'barbed wire disease'.

The phrase had been coined by Swiss physician Adolf Lukas Vischer who in 1918 published an account of the effect of incarceration on soldiers in the First World War. His book title was *Die Stacheldrahtkrankheit* and his English version *Barbed Wire Disease* was published a year later. In his studies, Vischer found that men who had been held captive as POWs for two years or more were more likely to suffer from mental illness, including an inability to concentrate, restlessness and having no interest in life.

Vischer had not been simply writing theories. He had witnessed these traits first hand having visited hundreds of prisoners of war in person with the Italian Red Cross. Although his book was groundbreaking in that it gave a name to a condition POWs felt during their incarceration, many experts still debated furiously whether 'barbed wire disease', or 'shell-shock', or any other of the host of terms to describe what returning soldiers and prisoners might be feeling even existed at all.

## THE TRAUMA OF CAPTIVITY

But the real prisoners of war themselves were also recording, writing, journaling and even writing poetry about how they were feeling as POWs. Writing, it seemed, would become a great outlet for the feelings of prisoners of war who felt they could not always talk about their experiences.

Archibald Allan Bowman was such a man. Bowman was a Scottish poet and philosopher and had been teaching at Princeton University when the world declared war in 1914. He returned to the United Kingdom a year later, enlisted and joined the Highland Light Infantry. He fought for three years but it was during the battle of Lys and Escaut in November 1918 that he was captured and taken to Rastatt prison camp in Baden, Germany. He wrote:

> Within these cages day by day we pace the bitter shortness of the meted span; and this and that way variously we plan our poor excursions over the poor place, cribbed to extinction. Yet remains one grace. For neither bars nor tented wire can ban full many a roving glance that dares to scan the roomy hill, and wanders into space. Yea, and remains for ever unrepealed and unimpaired the free impetuous quest of the mind's soaring eye, at length unsealed to the full measure of a life possessed awhile, but never counted, now revealed inestimable, wonderful, unguessed.

Bowman's writing is moving, detailed and yet, at times, curiously hopeful. After his capture he returned to the UK but was changed utterly by his incarceration. In his civilian life, he began delivering talks on adult furthering of education and became an avid supporter of the new League of Nations. The League, which was formed in 1919 as a direct response to the First World War, and whose aim was to maintain world peace, was something Bowman felt very strongly about.

## PSYCHOLOGICAL INTERVENTION

During his time as a POW, Bowman had written letters – often censored by his captors – to his wife Mabel. The letters are touching, often written as 'Daddy' to his children, talking of how he missed them, but also discussing the things he felt starved of as a prisoner: not only food but newspapers, education, socialising. To fill this intellectual gap, he spent his days running classes teaching his fellow captives German and even philosophy. This was a man who was used to lecturing the highest minds of university society but now he was lecturing the most basic, sometimes illiterate soldiers in a camp. But he was pleasantly surprised at how intelligent the soldiers were, saying he found soldiers: 'a splendid audience' and that he enjoyed lecturing them 'immensely'.

'Altogether my relations with the rank and file are extraordinarily happy. When at the end of a lecture I put questions, the men respond with eagerness and intelligence that would surprise you,' he wrote. It is clear that Bowman found writing – both his poetry and letters home – a great balm during a difficult time. But he seems to also have gained great peace and comfort from lecturing and teaching people such as the lowest ranking soldiers, people he would never have met or crossed paths with in normal civilian life. This 'purpose', this feeling of being needed, respected and useful in the horrors and ennui of a prisoner of war camp was surely what helped keep Bowman sane and able to carry on. But even that would end abruptly. In one letter he had written to his wife:

> I was suddenly ordered off without a moment's warning, had just time to shove my belongings into my pockets and go. The camp here is a small one and is situated on a very lovely and melancholy plain.[7]

Bowman survived being a prisoner of war and came home. It is no surprise that when he returned to civilian freedom he became a passionate supporter of the League of Nations, the organisation whose job it was to promote and maintain future peace. He wrote speeches and travelled, giving talks extolling the League of Nations. It appeared this POW used his experience to promote the 'good' that could come out of war, of lessons learnt and of the promise that nothing like this should ever happen again.[8]

Bowman died in 1936 aged only 53. His legacy included the sonnets written in captivity during the war, which he later said stood between 'my soul and madness', but also his moving letters to his beloved wife Mabel which were recorded. Their prose is romantic, loving and wistful and the reader can sense the happiness of their marriage. Although his death was untimely he was able to fill his last years with a purposeful vocation, of spreading the positive message of the League of Nations. Perhaps his happy marriage and support at home stopped him – like so many other ex-prisoners of war – from dwelling overly on what he had experienced, pushing him into forcing change for good from what he had gone through?

But at the heart of Bowman's mental survival after being held captive, was his urge to do something and to be active both morally, mentally and physically. This idea of keeping returning soldiers active rather than lamenting what they had been through was at the core of many lunatic asylums and their treatment plan for ex-prisoners of war. Many asylums extolled exercise, fresh air, keeping busy and not dwelling on what they had been through as the best ways of moving forward. But for many soldiers this was not enough. Shell-shock, which had started as a phrase to describe something no one really understood, was now being bandied about with alarming regularity. So much so that in 1922, the War Office Committee of Enquiry into 'Shell-Shock' was held. The Committee, made up of military and naval officers as well as leading eminent neurologists, were there to consider 'the different types of hysteria'.[9]

The aim was to investigate shell-shock and discuss whether the term should be used, or whether it was an accurate depiction of a mental illness or nervous condition at all. They concluded that the term shell-shock was 'a gross and costly misnomer which should be abolished', and that the war produced 'no new nervous disorders, but, owing to special conditions, the disorders produced appeared in some cases in aggravated form'.[10]

The committee decided that there were still only three main classes of disorder: genuine concussion as a result of a shell explosion, emotional shock, or nervous and mental exhaustion. They decreed that any type of person might suffer from one or all three of these conditions in modern warfare but that it was difficult to say beforehand 'what type of man is most likely to break down'.[11]

The resounding message from the Committee was this: that 'certain individuals' were unlikely to ever become efficient fighting soldiers but that training was key as well as morale, belief in the cause and that a man 'is part of the corporate whole'.[12]

The Committee also found that, in the large majority of cases of 'shell-shock', there was 'in the family or personal history evidence of weakness of instability of the nervous system'. This sweeping comment reflects the societal norms of the time – that if men could not overnight become soldiers and were in any way shocked emotionally, physically or mentally from the suffering they witnessed, then there must be a 'weakness' behind it all. Even more tellingly, they found that cowardice was, by definition, 'a lack of self-control in the presence of danger'.

With this kind of talk from the powers that be, it is little wonder that returning soldiers and ex-prisoners of war received virtually no help to reintegrate into society.

It is important to also include class in how we look at the treatment and subsequent mental health of prisoners of war. In many camps during the First World War, officers held captive were exempt from hard labour whereas the lower-class soldiers – privates, gunners and so on – were forced into physical work. Officers, on the whole, were also provided with better living conditions than lower-rank prisoners and were even assigned orderlies to make their beds and clean their clothing. Lower-rank soldiers on the other hand were forced to work for nothing or were given camp coupons – the currency of the camp. Ordinary soldiers' camps were composed of barracks made of wood which held around 250 prisoners each. Men slept on straw or sawdust and there would have been a small stove. A 3-metre high barbed wire fence surrounded the camps.

The one camp a soldier did not want to end up in was a reprisal camp. Situated usually in the coldest, most uncomfortable areas or near the battlefields, these camps made prisoners' lives hell. So called reprisal camps were designed to put pressure on opposing governments to release prisoners or for better treatment. But reprisal camps were also where prisoners who had attempted to escape were often sent as punishment. Here, men did not even sleep indoors on straw, but in makeshift tents resting on mud. Hard labour was replaced with the task of bringing back or burying corpses from nearby battlefields at the Front. Many prisoners of war in reprisal camps died there.[13] The cruelty in reprisal camps is difficult to comprehend. Word reached home of these camps and they were widely reported in national and local British newspapers:

> About March 1917 a 'reprisal' cage, about sixty yards square, was constructed by the Germans at a place called l'aviation on the road from Le Cateau to Wassigny. This was surrounded by an iron railing and was guarded by two sentries. By way of shelter from the weather, the prisoners, two in number, were accommodated in a very small hut about half a yard high and three feet long which did not permit of the whole of their bodies being covered. The prisoners were changed every twenty-one days and this 'reprisal camp' was in existence for four months. During that time it was quite impossible for the civilians to assist these prisoners. A Mdlle Druon Raymonde was able, for a little while, to pass them food by stealth but unfortunately she was detected and sent to prison.[14]

## PSYCHOLOGICAL INTERVENTION

Reprisal camps were places of terror because they were supposed to arouse a response in the opposing government, to instil a fear that any act of supposed aggression towards the belligerent state would be met with reprisals on their soldiers. Prisoners sent to them would have received the worst treatment, the worst food – if any – a lack of shelter, no warm or clean clothes and insufficient water.

> At Le Quesnoy, the Huns had what was called a reprisal camp which consisted of one open space enclosed with barbed wire. Squads of prisoners were driven into this place, where their already inadequate rations were still further reduced, and where they were kept without anything in the way of covering and in bitterly cold weather for periods extending to a fortnight. Complaints with regard to this inhumane treatment brought the retort that these were reprisals for the cruelty which was being meted out to German prisoners in Britain. In a company of about sixty prisoners who were thus kept in captivity for four days and four nights, half a dozen died from hunger and exposure.[15]

Far from hiding what went on in reprisal camps, the German government wanted the British government and British public to know just how bad the treatment was in a bid to damage British morale and encourage the British government to acquiesce to their demands. Unusually, they allowed prisoners to write of how badly they were being treated, allowed reporters to report on their treatment and even announced declarations, such as this:

> Curious proclamation from a German reprisal camp: A full copy of a proclamation read out to the British prisoners in a German reprisal camp near Lille is in possession of Private W.T. Owen, one of the three soldier sons of Mr Evan Owen, in Merthyr.

## THE TRAUMA OF CAPTIVITY

At Lille, in May 1917, 700 British prisoners were herded together, 350 in each of two parts of a dungeon-like place. They had only standing room on the first day, when they were kept without any food or drink. On each of the following six days each, fourteen men were given one 2lb loaf of German war bread, supplemented by some nauseating 'soup' which they were expected to drink out of their own steel helmets. They were avowedly punished as a 'reprisal' upon the British government and a German read out to them a 'declaration' on the subject. This stated:

Declaration to the English prisoners of respite. Upon the signal to withdraw the German prisoners of war to a distance of not less than 30km from the front line the British government has not replied. Therefore, it has been decided that all prisoners of war who will be taken in future will be held as prisoners of respite, i.e. very short of food, bad lodgings, no beds, hard work, also beside the German guns under shell-fire, no pay, no soap for washing or shaving, no bath, no towels or boots, etc. The English prisoners of respite are allowed to write to their relatives or persons of influence in England how badly they are treated.[16]

Away from the horror of reprisal camps, other camps had cultural spaces such as libraries, with books donated in parcels. In 1914, one camp in Munsigen received 220 books from the Red Cross. Newspapers, however old, were also delivered.

Officers, of course, would be more literate than the average private or working-class soldier, more likely to keep an eloquent diary, to be able to put their feelings into words, and to have access to books to read. Generally, rank and file soldiers would have been less able to commit their feelings to paper, something psychiatrists today say

## PSYCHOLOGICAL INTERVENTION

is an important part of acknowledging feelings, worries or doubts. Journaling or keeping a diary is often recommended today for those who are anxious, or have experienced trauma or mental illness. For the illiterate or sub-literate rank and file soldier, writing would not have – on the whole – been a consideration. Therefore working-class men were more likely to internalise trauma and stress, something which compounded their mental health problems further.

The result was, unsurprisingly, worse physical health at the end of the war, and worse mental health for lower-rank soldiers whose experience in camps would have been very different from that of officers. In Germany lice was so common among prisoners that by 1915, disinfection methods had to be put in place to de-lice soldiers' clothes and bedding. Typhus was also rife and at one camp, Totskoe in Russia, at least 10,000 men died.

Although a prisoner might have evaded illness, beatings or abuse, they are likely to have *witnessed* dreadful horrors. One such experience witnessed by other prisoners was the death of Able Seaman J.P. Genower, a prisoner of war at Brandenburg Camp, Germany. John Genower died as a result of 'burning', and the British government would later investigate his death. Other prisoners of war recounted what they saw:

> There was one hut apart from the others that served as a dungeon where they shut up prisoners who were rebellious. That day six Russians, one Frenchman and one Englishman were undergoing this punishment. Just against the hut there was a small workshop for repairs. Somebody had made a fire which had caught the timbers of the small prison. The prisoners noticed it and called out naturally to be let out, but in vain. The sentry remained unmoved. No doubt he was awaiting orders from his superiors. Those inside the dungeon were being choked. The Englishman broke the panes of a small window with

the idea of freeing himself and his companions. The sentry seeing him leaning out of the window gave him a tremendous bayonet thrust in the chest. The wounded man fell like lead. A small but revolting struggle then took place. The prisoners attempted to get out, and the German soldier reddened his bayonet again and again with the blood of the men shut up, who saw with horror that the fire was increasing. The conflagration could not be extinguished by the other prisoners until it had done its work. The eight unhappy individuals who had occupied the dungeon were corpses.[17]

The subsequent investigation into the death of John Genower and his fellow soldiers heard that Russian prisoners made the coffins for the burned men. They were buried in the cemetery at the Brandenburg prison camp. The investigation and witness statements of other prisoners makes for upsetting reading. One witness claimed the German sentry was unable to let the prisoners out for fear of not being given orders by his superiors. One prisoner, whose surname was Bates, had grabbed a large hatchet with which 'a few strong blows would have smashed the sides in' but had not been allowed to use it. Instead, the other prisoners of war were forced to stand there, watching their comrades burn to death and hearing their screams.[18]

This is just one of of the countless atrocities that occurred in prison camps during the Great War, but it serves as an example of how it wasn't always what a prisoner himself endured that would mark his mental health and emotional wellbeing forever, but bearing witness to the cruelty, abuse and murder of others.

Back at home in Britain psychiatrists had never seen 'shell-shock' or traumatic stress on this level and so there were many discussions on how it should be treated. The persistent notion that it didn't exist, or was just another form of 'hysteria' or cowardice, meant that many men did not receive even basic help.

## PSYCHOLOGICAL INTERVENTION

One man who did believe in shell-shock was psychiatrist Charles Myers. So disillusioned was he with how soldiers with shell-shock had been received and treated, that he refused to give evidence at the 1922 inquiry into shell-shock. Myers had been appointed by the Army during the war as part of the British Expeditionary Force to gather data on shell-shock and the rapidly increasing number of soldiers returning from the front with mental health difficulties.

The first cases Myers dealt with were physical difficulties such as hearing loss or tremor and headache. But he was quick to point out these were of a psychological origin rather than physical. He soon realised that soldiers were trying to suppress their feelings of fear and trauma and was one of the first to recognise that soldiers might only be 'cured' if they could re-live and talk about their experience. In other words, he believed in re-exposing them to the traumatic memories or events.

Myers advised the army of this and was allowed to set up four specialist units in 1916 but these were overwhelmed with casualties after the Battle of Arras and Passchendaele and his critics used this to retort that shell-shock was not a psychological disorder but merely cowardice. Myers returned to Britain in autumn 1917 where he saw that many soldiers returning with shell-shock were unable to hold down jobs and he managed to persuade the War Office to set up training courses for military psychiatrists for the treatment of shell-shock. But still, most wanted to believe shell-shock was cowardice or non-existent.

As such, many brutal treatments began to be used, one of which was electro-shock therapy. Respected neurologist Edgar Adrian was appointed to devise an electrotherapeutic treatment for soldiers with shell-shock. The therapy became incredibly popular in Britain – as well as in Europe – and involved a current being applied to body parts to 'cure' the symptoms. Often the electric current was applied directly to the body part causing problems, so for headache the current was applied to the head, for sudden mutism, the current was applied to the throat and for a man who could not walk, the electrical current was applied to the spine. Another therapy was exposure therapy where a soldier who feared being alone would be suddenly placed in isolation, or a soldier who feared the noise of shells was placed in a hospital room on a loud road to disturb his every waking moment.

Lewis Yealland was another doctor who believed in electroshock therapy. Canadian-born, he had moved to London during the Great War to work with paralysed soldiers and epileptics. He vocalised his belief that he did not believe shell-shock to be an illness, instead saying that men who claimed to be suffering from it lacked a sense of duty and discipline. Yealland was feared by many of his patients, and several of them decided to discharge themselves because they feared the treatment. One 35-year-old soldier, known as 'Frederic O', who had been paralysed in his lower limbs after a shell had exploded at Ypres, chose to discharge himself after having a nightmare in which he recounted seeing a white table and two dressing trolleys in a room painted white.

> On the floor were yards and yards of cable, which was strewn all over the place, and connected to a telegraph instrument placed upon an ordinary deal table. The room was crowded with nurses who were in white dresses and white aprons, they were all talking excitedly. A Doctor now enters in a white coat, he walks round the room, stepping over the coils of wire and is also excited and in a great hurry. He has a knife in his hand. ... The doctor was an exact representation of Dr Yealland.[19]

Although Yealland was feared by many patients, he claimed a 100 per cent success rate with his therapy. Yet his contemporary Dr Edgar Adrian later concluded that electric shock therapy was only able to remove motor symptoms – the cognitive and mental trauma remained. In a speech he conceded that there was obviously

## PSYCHOLOGICAL INTERVENTION

something else wrong and that the removal of the 'bodily symptom has not been enough'.

From a modern viewpoint it seems absurd that a doctor could believe a great trauma which causes a tremor might be cured by an electric shock, or that sending a terrified man to an isolation room might cure his trauma of imprisonment during the war. But one has to regard these treatments in the context of the era in which they were being performed. Masculinity, a sense of duty, bravery, and British stiff-upper-lip are never more under the spotlight than in times of war. Even if a returning soldier or prisoner had the bravery to admit he suffered from 'shell-shock', those who were charged with his treatment would often not have accepted his explanations and simply recorded him as a coward or an 'hysteric'. This societal problem with talking about men's mental health on their return from war meant that the vast majority of soldiers and prisoners returning to civilian life didn't receive anything near the level of support or treatment they needed to go on and live even a basic and content life.

The newspapers of the time did report shell-shock, but not in terms of understanding it or its origins. Instead, the term mostly appears in court cases where men 'used' shell-shock as a mitigating factor for a crime. In Glasgow an ex-soldier James Miller admitted stealing £17 from a labourer's coat at the Salvation Army hostel where he worked as cleaner. He cited shell-shock as his mitigating factor. Local and national newspapers from the 1917 into the 1920s cite court reports in which shell-shock was used as a defence for everything from violence to drink, from theft to bigamy. So much so that Doctor Hamblin-Smith, in a report to the Commissioners of Prisons, said: 'Shell-shock has taken the place of the "drink" excuse of my earlier years in the service. The estimation of the precise value of this excuse is a matter of great difficulty.'[20]

Relationships also inevitably came under strain when prisoners of war returned home. After being held captive many married soldiers, or soldiers who were engaged or courting, had not seen or heard from their women for months or even years. Some deserted their wives and these cases ended up before the courts. Some men became violent. In one case an ex-prisoner of war stood over his wife with a razor on his return but in his defence he said he had dreamt of her infidelity:

> An ex-soldier who was summoned at Sheffield Police Court for wife desertion told of a dream he had while he was a prisoner in Turkey. He stated that he dreamed he saw his wife in the company of a man. 'After I returned home I went with my wife to a swimming gala and there saw the man of my dream. My wife then admitted that she had been out with the man three times, the first occasion being on the night of my dream.' The wife denied that she had misconducted herself and said her husband had stood over her with a razor and extorted confessions from her. A separation order was granted.[21]

Of course, not every prisoner of war who returned suffered as badly as others might have. Some soldiers did indeed claim to be cured after treatment. One such soldier was Sergeant Wallace of the Royal Fusiliers:

> Treatment of shell-shock: Speech recovered by singing 'Roses of Picardy'. Singing is an important factor in the treatment of shell-shock at the Fourth London General Hospital, Denmark Hill, especially in cases of loss of speech.
> 'I attribute my cure to the singing of Roses of Picardy,' said Sergeant Wallace, late of the Royal Fusiliers whose speech was badly affected after he had been blown up in France. 'Before I started singing it used to take me about five minutes to get out my name and number but now I can talk quite well.'[22]

## PSYCHOLOGICAL INTERVENTION

Just after the war, 80,000 British soldiers had been treated for shell-shock-type neuroses. War pensions were given to 65,000 men for neuroses related to their war experience in the year of 1921. Eight years later, by 1929, over 47,000 men were in receipt of a pension for neurasthenia (chronic headaches, pain and fatigue.)[23]

Singing – however enjoyable or powerful a treatment for mutism – would not save the minds and souls of the thousands of prisoners of war whose experiences would haunt them for life. But, still, this had been the 'war to end all wars' and could never be repeated. That's what everyone told themselves. And although there might be a whole generation of men whose minds were damaged forever, this would surely never happen on this scale again.

# Chapter Four

# Prisoners of War in Germany – Second World War

'I have lived with prisoners of war from all ranks, of all the services, from all European fronts. On their behalf I resent any implication that they are below average in the qualities of balance, steadiness, patience, perseverance, tolerance or good humour.'

Major Charters, prisoner of war

'At the present moment the return of the prisoner, as distinct from that of the fighting man, has secured a dramatic hold on the public mind. The surge of Allied armies on German soil from east and west makes this irresistible. As liberation draws near, it throws into bold outline the drama of those long years in captivity. It makes the modern prisoner of war one with the age-long wanderer and exile who comes back to a world he scarcely knows and which scarcely knows him.'

British Prisoner of War Relatives' Association, no 58, February 1945

The low-rise buildings were surrounded by tall trees that cast leafy shadows onto cool glades beneath them. It was a place of peace, of safety. Children's laughter rang out as footsteps ran to and fro through the trees or, later, you might hear the sound of song around campfires. Stalag IX-B had been built just before the First World War to house German troops who trained in the area. During the war itself, the camp became a hospital town for wounded soldiers but now, in 1921, the camp was rented by the Kindererholungsstätte Wegscheide and the barracks were converted into summer camp residences for children. Each summer groups of children would stay here, enjoying the wide open space, the trees, the outdoors. But in 1939, the summer camp was suddenly closed and the Wehrmacht – the defence power forces of the Third Reich – impounded the area. Suddenly children's camp no more, the barracks were prepared to house soldiers once again and was renamed as Stalag IX-B.

Britain declared war on Germany on 3 September 1939 following Hitler's invasion of Poland. The same day, British Parliament immediately passed a bill imposing conscription on all men aged 18-41 – this was called the National Service Armed Forces Act. Many of these conscripted soldiers would have had fathers who had fought in the First World War, many of whom might not have returned home and some who might have been prisoners of war. Enforced conscription reflected this – many men would not have signed up voluntarily after seeing what their fathers went through twenty years earlier.

As the Second World War progressed, Stalag IX-B camp would house prisoners of war from eight countries including France, Russia, Italy, Britain, Serbia, Belgium, Slovakia and, later, the United States. By 1941, the camp housed over 18,000 prisoners. It was said that Soviet prisoners of war were treated the worst and by Christmas 1941 around twenty Soviet soldiers were dying per day. The camp was notoriously over-crowded and by 1942, so many prisoners were dying per day that the authorities dispensed with even issuing death certificates because they couldn't keep up.

Daily life for prisoners of war at Stalag IX-B was hard labour, including quarrying. But again, Soviet prisoners were given harder labour than other soldiers and were not even given shelter to sleep beneath. At the same time, the systematic genocide of millions of

## THE TRAUMA OF CAPTIVITY

Jews was happening and Nazi captors had worked out the most effective ways of killing through work before killing by gas. Although incomparable to the Holocaust, in German POW camps captors were also becoming well-versed in systematic, organised cruelty.

As in the First World War, most British officers in German prisoner of war camps were treated with a level of decency. Germany had, after all, signed up to the Geneva Convention and vowed to adhere to its treatment of prisoners of war. Through the use of cinema newsreels, radio news and the improved technology used by newspaper companies, news of prisoners of war returned to the UK at a much faster rate than during the First World War.

Prisoners of war were often spoken about with reverence – particularly the 'bad boys' who regularly attempted to escape and were ultimately sent to Colditz – where the escapees from other prisoner of war camps were sent as a last resort. Colditz, infamous and the subject of many films, was a twelfth-century castle set on a rock in Colditz, south of Leipzig. Its inmates included notables such as Viscount Lascelles, who was also nephew of King George VI. With his royal connections, the viscount was considered one of the 'prominente' at Colditz because he could be used as a potential bargaining chip by the Nazis should they need to.

One prisoner was Malcolm McColm who had been sent to Colditz after escaping from other German prison camps. When interviewed for a newspaper on his return, McColm said that of the four camps he had endured, Colditz held the most 'lively' memories where he mingled with Dutch, French, Belgians and Yugoslavians and told the reporter that 'each nation vied with the others to see who could annoy the Germans the most.'[1]

This fighting British, stiff-upper-lip spirit was reported time and again in the UK press, particularly in reference to Colditz which, despite being a place regular escapees were sent was, on the whole, a place where prisoners were treated with relative respect. In fact, the recurrent escapees sent to Colditz were often more prone to trying to escape from there than anywhere else.

One of the most incredible escape stories is told by Lieut. Steven Wright, of the 9th Lancers, youngest son of Captain and Mrs H. FitzHerbert of Yeldersley Hall who is home after five years in captivity in numerous German prison camps. He made five separate bids for freedom and his most bitter recollection is of the occasion when he was within a stone's throw of the Dutch border and was betrayed – by a rainstorm!

Lieut. Wright and a brother officer 'started a racket' by pretending they were suffering from nervous disorders. 'Drinking a lot of strong coffee to keep ourselves alert, we did our stuff before a mixed commission and ten days later we were sent to a lunatic asylum, south west of Dortmund,' states Lieut. Wright. 'This institution was extremely efficient and well run and I have nothing but admiration for the way we were treated. But unfortunately they took away our clothes and shoes every night so there was nothing for it but to escape in our pyjamas!'[2]

Lieutenant Wright escaped from the asylum with his comrades and took maps and compasses. They slept in cornfields by day and travelled by night and spent eleven nights walking until they reached the Dutch border. Just when they were in sight of the border, however, a rainstorm broke out which masked the noise of Germans hiding nearby who ambushed them and returned them back to Colditz. These plucky, positive stories were reaching home in droves and so rather than dwell on the misery of being held captive in a German prison camp, the public might have been forgiven for believing that being a prisoner of war was a little like a game, a challenge, full of camaraderie, of daring escape plans all under the perplexed gaze of seemingly forgiving and indulgent German captors.

## THE TRAUMA OF CAPTIVITY

But as Lieutenant Wright explained in another more thoughtful interview with the press, the monotony of daily life in Colditz did take its toll on his mental health.

> 'It was the monotony which drove men mad [...] The walls in this old castle, [...] which was built in 1300 and in turn had been, in modern times, a concentration camp, lunatic asylum, and even a home for fallen girls, seemed to be impregnated with the misery of the countless occupants, who had been the victims of some form of brutality or other and it was this uncanny atmosphere and its associations which affected them more than any physical torture.'[3]

Lieutenant Wright went on to explain that after one of his many escape attempts, he was told he would be shot by the Gestapo, before being placed in solitary confinement in a cell of only 13ft by 9ft – where he stayed for five months. In the same interview, Wright explained that a German general had visited him in his small cell and apologised for the treatment he had received by the Gestapo.

> I was by that time a sorry sight, very emaciated and weak and the German general promised me that I should be sent to a convalescent home. However the whole camp was sent to a reprisal camp in Poland because we were told German officers who were prisoners of war in Canada were being treated badly.[4]

Reprisal camps, it seemed, were used on anyone – ordinary soldier, bad boy escapee of Colditz – for Germany to score points with its enemy. Another returning prisoner of war was Colonel German who had been held in prisoner of war camps in Germany for five years. On his arrival he told waiting press: 'I am very glad to be home. Five years is a long time.'

## PRISONERS OF WAR IN GERMANY – SECOND WORLD WAR

But again, read on in the interview and it is revealed that the mental side of the experience was worse for him than anything physical he had endured:

> The physical side of the experience [...] one could put up with, it was the mental side that was difficult. The boredom and monotony were the worst and he paid a great tribute of appreciation to the people of Leicester and Leicestershire for the way they had supported the fund run by his wife for the benefit of Leicestershire prisoners and that had played a big part in helping the mental side.[5]

His wife had organised local people to prepare parcels of food and clothing to be sent to prisoners of war in Germany. All over Britain, other groups, particularly women's groups, were doing the same. Parcels would become a great source of comfort to captured soldiers in Germany. The Red Cross sent out parcels containing items such as butter, chocolate, condensed milk and biscuits, comparatively luxurious to the two meals a day of black bread and soup most prisoners of war existed on.

Parcels were of enormous importance to men's morale not only because they helped them survive physically – but because parcels were a symbol of home, a reminder that others were thinking of them, that they had not been forgotten. Women's groups such as the Women's Institute were hugely active in providing such care parcels for prisoners in Germany. They knitted pullovers for prisoners of war as well as providing so called 'occupational parcels', which included examples and patterns for things prisoners could make such as tea cosies, fire screens and bags as well as gloves and belts.

For those returning from German prisoner of war camps, society welcomed them on the whole as heroes. In fact, to return as a prisoner of war from Germany – particularly if one had attempted to escape – was seen as a great feather in the cap of many soldiers. So much so that many con artists posed as escapee prisoners of war to be paid to do public talks. One such con artist was 34-year-old George Edward Bernard Hayward. He had been a private in the war but posed as a sergeant major who had escaped from a German prisoner of war camp. He travelled around Rotherham, Manchester and Liverpool dressed in a sergeant major's uniform, giving talks of his POW camp exploits in cinemas. He'd even chartered a private plane to take him from talk to talk. He was finally arrested by police when he stole money from two women – one of whom had put him up for the night as a hero.[6]

Hayward was sentenced to twelve months' hard labour for theft and his cover was blown. But it is telling how the public reacted to the heroes who had been prisoners of war, particularly those who had daring tales of escape to tell. Lauded as heroes, these men received warm welcomes and paying customers to hear their stories. One real ex-prisoner of war who gave talks was Reverend H. Burns Jamieson who had been a padre in prisoner of war camps in Germany. He gave talks to the public, which he began by saying: 'This is not a subject on which I am very fond of talking. It is something one has tried to forget, although not the lessons that one has learnt from it.'

Reverend Jamieson had been captured in 1942 in North Africa and taken prisoner of war by the Germans. In his speech he conceded that he took comfort from his faith and being allowed to pray while taken prisoner, but he added:

> there was a strain due to the lack of freedom and food and also there seemed no point in doing things. Overcrowding was also hard to bear and you could never cross the room without having to ask someone to move. There was a sense of loneliness and a strain due to the news on the radio. Constant searches of the huts were made by the Germans.[7]

Indeed, the monotony, loneliness and depression many of these men felt were often eclipsed in the news of the day of the daring feats of escape of other prisoners. Perhaps it was easier and more pleasant for the public to look on these men as plucky heroes rather than damaged souls who still had so many terrible memories of incarceration.

One such story was that of Walter Charles Dark, aged 30, who was found dead at the bottom of a cliff in Devon in 1946. Dark had joined the Army in 1939 and had been captured by the Germans at Mersa Matruh in 1941. He was then taken as prisoner of war where he remained for four years until the end of the war.

After Walter's body was found, his father Charles told an inquest that:

> since his son's return he had periodic fits of depression and nervousness and last December on the advice of Dr Lees had entered Axminster Hospital, whence he returned home on January 30th, when, though generally normal, he still seemed worried about a claim he had made for a pension.[8]

It was becoming apparent in newspaper reports, interviews with returning prisoners of war and in the field of psychology, that how a man dealt with being a prisoner was not only down to what he endured, but how his own pre-conditioned mind dealt with that – upbringing, experience, previous depressive personality, strong family ties or no family ties – all had an influence over how a prisoner of war would deal with his experiences.

One such example is that of the famous 'legless' RAF flying ace Wing Commander Douglas Bader. A double amputee, Bader joined the RAF as the first and only disabled person to fly with artificial legs. When his Spitfire collided with another British plane, Bader had to parachute out and lost one of his artificial legs in the process. 'I had to jettison one of my legs. The thing caught and snapped off and I felt like a fool parachuting down with only one leg.'[9]

Bader was taken to a hospital, from which he escaped, but the Germans caught him. The RAF flew over and dropped him a replacement artificial leg but his captors would not let him have it. 'You know those goons wouldn't let me have my new leg for two weeks. Then they wanted to punish me for trying to escape.'[10]

In a rather light-hearted interview, Bader explained how it made him feel as a prisoner being robbed of his artificial leg. His tone is light and careless in interviews, but the humiliation he felt at being carried everywhere by his enemy as a prisoner is tangible:

> It was a magnificent example of how the German mind works. They wouldn't give me my legs. Two goons carried me while another officer marched along in front. I felt, without legs, like you would feel walking down Piccadilly without your pants. Everyone was staring and looking at me. One of the guards would stand at the bathroom door with a pistol drawn as though I'd walk off on my hands.[11]

Bader tried to escape his prison camp four times, even fashioning a glider with other inmates and trying to launch it from the camp roof. Each time he was captured but when asked why he kept doing it, he replied: 'That sounds silly to you people who've been outside but to those of us inside, it was because any means of escape was better than sitting around doing nothing.'

Bader explained in interviews that his hatred of his captors and his own refusal to do as they said kept him going.

> We were like schoolkids with men's minds [...] We would refuse to do anything until they pulled a pistol and then we would smile and obey orders. We baited them all the time. The only thing that saved us was a sense of humour. The German has no sense of humour and if you laugh at him he thinks his honour is involved. That's why we could enrage them so easily.[12]

But not every returning prisoner of war would have Douglas Bader's mental strength. That was to be the problem surrounding returning prisoners of war – they were so very different from returning soldiers. But they were also different among themselves. How would they reintegrate back into society? The British Prisoners of War Relatives' Association published a regular magazine for its members. In an issue from February 1945, the association talked of the 'problem' of the returning prisoner of war.

> At the present moment the return of the prisoner, as distinct from that of the fighting man has secured a dramatic hold on the public mind. The surge of Allied armies on German soil from east and west makes this irresistible. As liberation draws near, it throws into bold outline the drama of those long years in captivity. It makes the modern prisoner of war one with the age-long wanderer and exile who comes back to a world he scarcely knows and which scarcely knows him.[13]

This was still months before the end of the war, but people were rightly already anticipating that the returning prisoner was very different to the returning soldier. A prisoner had been in the war – but not *in* the war. He had endured the years of war, but not the fighting after being held captive. His battle had been with his own mind, his hunger, his survival and other internalised thoughts, as well as any physical brutalities he might have endured. The Relatives' Association rightly focused on how the prisoner might feel on his return, not on how society ought to feel about him.

> Thousands of prisoners of war know nothing of rationing of any sort. They are unaware of the revolution wrought in the home by the servant problem, the disappearance of the car, the shortage of fuel, the inability to repair and renew household goods. They have no knowledge

of the mental and emotional upheaval caused by long evacuation, by the damage of one house in three all over Britain by enemy raids. They do not know how five years have broken ties and changed friendships and destroyed settled habits and created new ways of daily life.[14]

Indeed, post-war Britain would have been a shock for anyone returning from war, but particularly so to a man who had been imprisoned. Many men wrote that their dreams of home kept them going, dreams of seeing their streets or town, their houses, the locations they knew well. Many of these had now been bombed or experienced major damage from shelling and did not look as the men had left them. Rationing – which would go on long after the war – would mean that returning prisoners would not get to eat the food they had dreamt of while on starvation rations in camps. A home, good food, normal life – all this would have changed while they were away. To return to something so different from the memories that had kept them going would no doubt be a huge shock and a grave disappointment. But one man – Major Charters – a doctor who was taken prisoner of war in Greece while fighting in 1941, believed that returning prisoners of war would not be 'a problem', although he conceded many had suffered mental tortures that would last a lifetime. He responded to a letter in the *British Medical Journal* in which a Dr Harkness described returning prisoners of war as 'problems for their lifetimes':

> I hope that interest in the prisoners of war will be sustained throughout the post-war years and that this time some sympathetic action will be taken. The cause of the men will need the powerful advocacy of the Press and people and the BMJ could play a leading part. Major Newman discusses the officer prisoner. The large majority of our prisoners are NCOs and men and the conditions will be sharply different from that experienced by the officers.

> I feel that Major Newman is too optimistic about early recovery ... the very large majority of our returning prisoners of war will be problems for their lifetime. The men on return will find the war over and be bewildered and hurt by public reaction and indifference. They should not be demobilised but offered a period of reasonable financial security. The alternative of attempting to assess disability and granting a pension will have to be considered. The establishment of prisoner of war clubs is likely, in my opinion, to retard rehabilitation. The returned prisoner should be encouraged to mix with others who have not suffered similar experiences and to merge as soon as possible into normal service or civil society ... John Harkness.[15]

Harkness's intentions were of course honourable. His concerns were echoed around Britain from the wives of returning prisoners of war, their children, their employers – no one knew how to react to the men when they came home. Should they treat them with kid gloves? Should they ask about their time in prison camps? Should they encourage talking? Or pretend it had not happened? John Harkness's letter to the BMJ echoed those worries and concerns and his remark that returning prisoners of war might well be 'problems for their lifetimes' was something every single person remotely linked to a POW was dreading. Could the employer take back such a damaged man? Could he be relied upon to do his old job as he had before the war? Could the wife sleep at night next to a man who had suffered horrors that might lead him to call out in the night or even become violent? Should children run to their fathers and ask for cuddles, or leave him to his thoughts? These debates were going on in households both rich and poor and behind the closed doors of businesses all over the country. If the prisoner of war would be a problem for his lifetime, how on earth was society meant to cope?

# THE TRAUMA OF CAPTIVITY

On reading Harkness's letter in the *British Medical Journal*, Major Charters wrote a riposte from his incarceration in a prisoner of war camp – Stalag IX-B:

> No one realises more acutely than I do the pressing psychological problems which in certain cases have resulted from years of enforced idleness, of monotony, and of physical suffering and disablement. Nevertheless I must emphatically deny that anything approaching a majority of prisoners will be 'problems for their lifetime'. Rather I would say that the majority of these men have gained tolerance, understanding, patience, forbearance and courage.[16]

Major Charters's letter, written from the very camp where he had seen fellow prisoners of war with his own eyes and had, by his own admittance, seen how well connected they were as comrades and in community life, was an advocate of prisoners of war returning home and not being anticipated as problems for society.

He wrote:

> I have shown Dr Harkness's letter to several of the men here – cheerful, average, level-headed individuals. They expressed themselves as follows: 'Afraid he doesn't altogether know what he is talking about: a few special cases, yes, but not the very large majority!' By all means let us arrange for physical and mental rehabilitation where it is needed. By all means let us make some allowances for the fact that the average prisoner of war is not adjusted to the change of the last five years. But do not let us discuss the majority as if they were psychopathological problems. Above all, let us avoid discussing

> their 'mentality' in the lay press ... I have lived with prisoners of war from all ranks, of all the services, from all European fronts. On their behalf I resent any implication that they are below average in the qualities of balance, steadiness, patience, perseverance, tolerance or good humour. The average prisoner is not a 'problem' to himself, his companions or his future employer. Surely Dr Harkness takes a very pessimistic view of the mental and moral stamina of our race.[17]

The major had good intentions: he wanted to warn British society against a preconceived idea that all returning prisoners of war would be damaged, troubled, unable to slot back into their place or work or place in the family. He had seen first hand, he claimed, that men could survive being a prisoner of war without being overly damaged. But the newspapers were running stories of men returning home from camps who were recounting not only the cruelty but shame of being held prisoner of war. One such man was Private Jack Mitchell, 7th Battalion Royal Sussex Regiment who was a shop assistant before being called up and captured at Amiens and held in Stalag 20B.

Said the local paper:

> They lived on a starvation diet – he himself as been a stretcher case from lack of food and warmth – and but for the Red Cross parcels, which came as a godsend, he could not have survived. He has experienced all the cruelty of forced marches: foot gear gone and feet wrapped in sacking and two German guards to every three men. What he hated most was the propaganda march through Poland with a wireless van in the front and in the rear announcing at intervals: 'These are the men who laid down their arms and would not fight for Churchill!'

## THE TRAUMA OF CAPTIVITY

There were 5,000 prisoners of war and most of them were wounded or suffering with burns from mortar fire. If a man dropped out he was remorselessly shot by the guard. Once they were billeted in an underground fort, dank with stagnant water. During the three weeks they stayed there, eighty-five men died of starvation and diphtheria.[18]

The camaraderie and stoicism Major Charters might have witnessed in the camps were sure to be tested on the prisoners' return. Knowing your place in the camp is one thing. Returning and carrying on a life you left behind several years before was quite another. Psychoanalysts of the time knew this and were already working with returned prisoners of war who were damaged. Indeed, throughout the Second World War the most serious cases of mental disorder were sent to Northfield Hospital in Birmingham, also known as Hollywell Mental Hospital. Soldiers sent here were active fighters as well as escaped prisoners of war.

Psychoanalyst John Rickman began working at Northfield in July 1942 and was later joined by Wilfried Bion.

John Rickman was at the time one of the most revered psychoanalysts in Britain. Strangely, being put in charge of soldiers and prisoners of war, Rickman had been a conscientious objector. He had been analysed by Freud himself. The 'Crookham Experiment' was also a programme designed to rehabilitate returning soldiers and prisoners of war. This scheme, at the Royal Army Medical Corps depot in Crookham, ran from November 1943 to February 1944 and saw 1,200 prisoners of war go through a four-week course of rehabilitation. This was necessary because the British government were already labelling prisoners of war 'the awkward lot' because they so often returned with sickness – both physical and psychological.

These prisoners of war were reported to have severe 'stalag mentality' from their time in captivity and suffered from depression, guilt and anxiety.

## PRISONERS OF WAR IN GERMANY – SECOND WORLD WAR

Lieutenant-Colonel Tommy Wilson, was an army psychiatrist who had worked at the Tavistock Clinic. He published a report with recommendations on how returning prisoners of war should be received and treated on their return home. But it was not only thanks to Tommy Wilson that the plight of prisoners of war became more widely spoken about. As the Second World War dragged on, many respected ex-prisoners of war from the First World War wrote to the War Office explaining that something must be done for the current soldiers because they were still suffering from the psychological impact of captivity fifteen years on.

Tommy Wilson did not believe these men had psychiatric problems per se, but more that they were special cases – men who had been taken from one environment, forced to live in another during great hardship, and then returned to their original environment. Wilson wrote a nine-page report on the psychological aspects of the rehabilitation of repatriated prisoners of war. His work had a resounding effect in government and in time, approval was given for a new scheme: Civil Resettlement Units. These were units run by the army and government that would provide help and support in the progression from returning prisoner of war to ordinary civilian. Attendance was not obligatory and leaflets about the resettlement units were handed out to prisoners of war two weeks before their leave would begin.

As attending a CRU would be voluntary and at the discretion of the returning POW, organisers did their best to make the idea as appealing as they could, ensuring the resettlement units were as close as possible to the homes of the POWs. The organisers also deemed it particularly important that the units did not in any way resemble camp life as a prisoner of war. So, men of all ranks dined together at tables in the same dining hall. Instead of queueing for self-service meals, waiting staff were employed to serve the men at table – another differentiation from life as a prisoner of war men longed to forget. At weekends, men could go home and if they wanted could bring their wives and children to the unit to meet others like them.

## THE TRAUMA OF CAPTIVITY

When men wanted to share their feelings, they were encouraged to in an early form of group therapy. For those whose problems seemed greater, they could be referred to a psychiatrist with no shame. But even then, the emphasis was on voluntary help rather than being forced. For men who had been unable to return to work, the CRUs offered guidance and training in practical skills to find new work. These units carried on aiding returning men for two years until the spring of 1946 and at least 13 per cent of prisoners of war attended one. In a study by the Army, fifty men who had attended a CRU were compared with a hundred who had not and it was found that 74 per cent of ex-prisoners of war who had attended a resettlement unit were more settled.

As for Wifriend Bion, during the 1940s and as soldiers and prisoners of war began to return home, he began focusing more and more on group psychology. In 1946, he founded the Tavistock Institute at the Tavistock Clinic where he had worked since 1932 and would later write a paper called 'Experiences in Groups'. As discussed earlier in this book, Wilfred Bion had been a tank commander in the First World War (and narrowly missed being awarded a Victoria Cross because he swore at his superiors). At Tavistock men were mostly treated at first with sedatives but Bion wanted to remind the men who they were. He emphasised that they were still 'soldiers' not merely infirm or patients. He spoke to them of joining together as a band of brothers to fight in the 'battle' against neurosis.

Bion encouraged the men to do one hour's exercise a day in a group, but he was unconventional in that he did not seek to control or discipline them, instead letting them behave as they wished, allowing them to be as neurotic, loud, aggressive, emotional as they liked. When the men said they wanted to start a dancing class, Bion did not scoff but allowed them to organise it. During six weeks of unconventional therapy – allowing the returning soldiers to behave and express themselves as they wanted, but by being encouraged to do all this in a group – the men found that they began to self-organise themselves and find a morale together they did not have before. Bion went on to become Director of the London Clinic of Psychoanalysis and President of the British Psychoanalytical Society.

Another important aspect of returning prisoners was that of whether they had escaped or not. In a paper 'Neurosis in Escaped Prisoners of War', written by Manfred Jeffrey and E.J.G. Bradford in 1946, they studied forty soldiers who were escaped prisoners of war. These men had been referred because of neurosis and were 'truculent, suspicious, hostile and disinclined to discuss their condition'.[19]

The paper found that these men were insistent on being referred to as 'escaped prisoners of war' and not average soldier repatriates. Of interest was that thirty-six of the escaped prisoners of war were 'resentful about the circumstances of their capture' and stated that their capture was not their fault and was due to a blunder by someone else. The men were held in camps in Africa under Italian jailers and suffered diarrhoea of which many other men died. Bad sanitation and underfeeding led to 'lassitude, headache, loss of weight, poor concentration and depression'.[20]

This study discovered that these forty men found it harder to feel part of the group and as a result were more isolated. The men, when interviewed, said they had felt most anger not towards their captors but towards their NCOs and officers in their prisons who they felt had withheld food, deprived them of rations and been the gatekeepers of deciding who went on outdoor working parties. The study found that the prisoners' hatred of these authority or 'father' figures added to their anger and stress during their incarceration which would have been less had they felt assimilated into the group.

> Thoughts and impulses centred around escape were more prevalent than among prisoners of war generally. In a significant number it reached obsessional tension. The primitive aggressive function, the drive towards autonomy, to the complete mastery over the environment,

had to be satisfied even if only in fantasy. In fact, however, twelve men of our series made no fewer than thirty-two attempted escapes involving much risk. One man, a paratrooper, doing a considerable amount of killing in effecting his escapes.[21]

This study found that once escaped, the men had considerable difficulty maintaining their freedom. They wandered for ten months in 'loosely organised' smaller groups of four to five men. Some found places to hide in isolated farms, others in single rooms. Others relied on locals bringing food under cover of darkness. One of the men spent four months living in the hills alone, and while six men found their way to neutral Switzerland by the Armistice, two had had to make daring escapes from trains.

This study found that: 'Periods of depression, brooding, startle and terror dreams were common, especially in such men as witnessed the killings of comrades and hosts.' One man in particular in the study, described as a large man of the Jewish faith and who had lost his wife back in Britain during an air raid, had joined a guerrilla band and become their leader. 'His habit was to execute personally all captives. He experienced headaches and a peculiar feeling of tension, which eased somewhat after killing or fighting.'[22] This Jewish case study returned to Britain as an escaped POW but suffered from severe headaches and was said to suffer from bouts of aggression and depressive episodes.

The study found that on return to Britain, the men varied in their attitudes to authority figures. Bradford and Jeffrey wrote that some reacted with surprise that the Military Police were kind to them, however some of the returning escapees went absent saying that they did not worry about punishment after all they had been through. Of great interest was one area of the study which found that: 'They felt that the men regarded them as lucky "as if we had been loafing while they had been fighting".'

Thirty of the forty escaped POWs in this study admitted to feeling this way – that other soldiers might regard them as lesser beings because they had been 'loafing' in incarceration while soldiers fought the real war. These feelings only got worse as the men attempted to resettle into life at home. Some of the men said they felt people were 'not interested in their story', while others felt that strangers were laughing at them or making disparaging remarks. Twenty-eight of the men, according to the study, said they felt friends were strangers or enemies and that friends coming to the house were 'invaders' and three quarters of the men preferred to stay at home all day by the fireside with their eating habits altered: they swung between craving huge meals and having no appetite at all.

Relationships of course suffered and this study found that some of the men were now 'troubled' by homosexual fantasies since being incarcerated with only other men. Thirty-six of the forty men in the study said they were 'quarrelsome' within their relationships and the same number were now claustrophobic. Of major note in the study was this:

> One of the effects of imprisonment is social degradation; the prisoner realises that he belongs to an inferior class, he has less food, freedom and pleasure, he is deprived of a sex life, and of the amenities of his group and cultural pattern. Vis-à-vis his guard, he is an inferior.[23]

The study by Jeffrey and Bradford makes for fascinating reading even though it concerns only forty escaped prisoners of war. One line in particular stands out which is concerning the desire of most of the men in the study to eat at home rather than out at another person's house: 'The food was literally "home baked", and so they are absorbing the home back into themselves.'[24] This desire to eat large quantities, at home, made at home, probably served by a wife or mother figure, no doubt led the returning prisoner of war to feel great comfort, but followed often by feelings of anger and self-loathing at being 'dependent' once again just as they had felt in prison.

Studies and results from psychological experiments are one thing, but it was quite another to live with a returning prisoner of war in a day-to-day, non-clinical setting. Of course, these clinics and hospitals were very important and necessary for the analysis of returning prisoners of war and to aid them in discussing their own mental health, but while a man might be willing to discuss his experiences with other soldiers or a psychiatrist, he might be a very different man at home. So how was it for a family to take back a prisoner of war into their fold?

Lorna Doyle's father Dennis Brock was a prisoner of war in Germany during the Second World War. He endured horrors such as having to pick out body parts after the Allied bombing of the city of Dresden while he was a prisoner held nearby. But his daughter, although recalling some of his darker memories, has fond memories of him as a father.

## 'He talked about his time as a prisoner of war in schools'

Lorna Doyle, whose father Dennis Brock was a prisoner of war in Germany:

My father was Dennis Brock and he was called up right at the very beginning of the war. He had six months' training which all the young men about the age of 20 had before war was declared. Then they went back to their homes and when war was declared he was called up. After basic training at Harrogate from September 1939, he went to France and was rescued off the beaches of Dunkirk.

Then he went to Ascot racecourse for training then he was sent to the desert in North Africa. My dad was captured there in 1942 so he was a POW from 1942 to the end of the war – three years.

# PRISONERS OF WAR IN GERMANY – SECOND WORLD WAR

Italy was involved with North Africa at the time, so at first Dad and the other prisoners were transported to a POW camp in Italy. But once Italy changed its allegiance the POWs, including Dad, were taken to East Germany. They were transported in cattle trucks.

My father was taken to a labour camp and he and the other prisoners were sent out to work in brick fields. They did have some means of writing, basic things so they could write letters home and could receive them but all this was very disjointed. They wouldn't hear from anyone for six months then get a pile of letters. I've got letters from my parents to each other with many post marks. At that time my dad wasn't engaged to my mother. They'd been very good friends since early teens and it's rather touching because, as the war progressed when he came home on leave he realised it was developing into more than friendship. She felt the same and waited for him and they got engaged in 1945 when he came home.

My parents waited a year before they married cos they didn't want to get married before my mum's brother was demobbed and wanted the whole family back safely. As for my dad's time in the camps, they had a long working day, were marched off to the brick fields each day to work. The biggest, most awful thing was the bombing of Dresden in 1945. He was in Dresden in a POW camp and the next day the prisoners had to go into the cities and drag out the bodies of the civilians. While it was going on, he saw people exploding in front of him, terrible things. He'd talk about fireballs, and heat. One Christmas in the camp they were told they'd get a very special Christmas gift and food was on their minds. It turned out to be raw fish heads with the eyes in ... That was the sort of thing they had to put up with.

Looking at the photos I have of my father, he doesn't seem to have suffered emaciation but they all lost a lot of weight. From a healthy 11 stone he was down to about seven. In the years afterwards when he came home he suffered from skin eruptions and boils and shingles. When my parents married, the doctors advised him to keep chickens because of rationing and my dad needed food they couldn't get in plentiful supply. So my parents they kept chickens and a vegetable garden to get the food he needed.

Incredibly he had no stomach complaints but then he'd been very fit before the war with cycling. When he saw the family doctor when he came home the doctor said he wouldn't make old bones. But my father lived to be 101! It was remarkable.

My father had a cheerful attitude. You think how did he stay so cheerful? He had a very deep religious faith. All his life right up to the end – and I think that and the way he dedicated his life to the local church St Mary's kept him sane. The big issue for him was finding a settled job. He'd left school without any qualifications. Because of his disjointed upbringing – he was brought up by grandparents – he was not able to take up a grammar school place and had a secondary modern education and spent the early years of their marriage doing correspondence courses to upgrade his education.

He succeeded and got into the civil service which was considered a very secure, but not very well-paid, job.

In 1952, I was only 16 months old when Dad's father-in-law died very suddenly and the family just collapsed. Suddenly Dad had to take over and he was the one who kept everyone going. There were difficulties but his resilience shone through all the time. He did talk about being a POW with us a lot. My mother encouraged it. When he was home in 1945, Mum took Dad to the cinema. They'd always been great cinema goers and loved watching films. But it was a big mistake. He was sitting in the dark and it made him very, very uneasy. He wasn't ready to be in a place where he was uncomfortable, looking out for possible attacks. He realised that if he wanted to talk about it, it was good. The right thing not to bottle it up. He never did. So I was quite young when I found out. I was probably only about 7 because I told my teachers at school that my father had been in prison and my mother said you mustn't say that, it's a different kind of prison! So I was aware of it.

He brought back various medals and memorabilia. I think his talking helped him. He could talk about it easily with me. It was part of life, it happened. He talked about it as if it all happened yesterday. It was obviously very imprinted in his mind. There were some awful things. A young man was shot in front of them – a young American POW – for some perfectly trivial reason. They marched home in May 1945 and it was after the war had finished and they were walking through a forest to make their way to the Allies and one of their German guards hung on behind with his wife and son and begged them to take them to the Allies and my father realised he couldn't do that because a day or two before they'd been enemies. His nature was to say yes, But as a soldier, he couldn't say yes. That upset him.

As for support, there was no professional help. They were expected to pick up where they had left in 1939. He'd had a very hard upbringing. He'd lost his mother at the age of 5 and his father more or less gave him away to grandparents and he never saw his father again. Everywhere he was moved to he wrote to his father to say where he was but he never heard back. He was a village boy. There was no money with his grandparents. So anything he wanted he had to make. He was just a bit like a little scavenger but he latched onto St Mary's church and cycling and bellringing. But because of his tough start he wasn't pampered in any way and had no expectations of anything in life. He didn't feel hard done by in any way.

The army became a purpose and a new family for him in a way. My mother and her family provided the family he didn't have, and gave him access to things he'd yearned for such as nice music because of his disadvantaged upbringing. The letters from my mother during his time as a POW kept him going.

With me, my father was delightful. He was a serious father but he was lovely. Right up to the end you could always go to him with a problem. I don't remember him ever getting very cross with me. He left that to my mother! He was just there for me all the time. He was a very caring person.

# THE TRAUMA OF CAPTIVITY

In the last years of his life, Dad talked to schools about his time as a POW.

My father died July 2020 aged 101. It's strange to think now that when he was a prisoner he didn't see my mother for four years. But when he came back he was so well-adjusted and just a wonderful man. I realise how lucky we were now.

Dennis Brock's case was a happy one and his daughter can only recall his kindness, which proves that not all men were damaged by being a prisoner of war. John Procter was another British man who was taken prisoner in Germany. His daughter, Mandy Procter, said he had a great many mental health problems and nightmares when he returned.

## 'Dad was in and out of hospital and couldn't hold jobs down'

Mandy Procter, daughter of John Procter who was prisoner of war in Germany for five years:

My father John was captured in France in April 1940. He was a tank driver and they got attacked and captured and he went through a number of POW camps because they moved them around to different stalags. They were put in working squads and they'd work in mines and quarries. My father was only 19 at the time.

My dad's brother was also in the forces and his wife happened to work with a lady and he asked if she'd like to write to my dad as a pen pal while he was in the camp. She did, and that's how they got to know each other. The lady would become my mother. Dad was called John but everyone called him Jack. He began writing to my mother and through their letters they fell in love. He wrote to her of how he was longing to meet her, to get home and hopefully become romantically involved. I think the letters must have kept him going.

He was held as a prisoner for four years and 364 days – just one day short of five years.

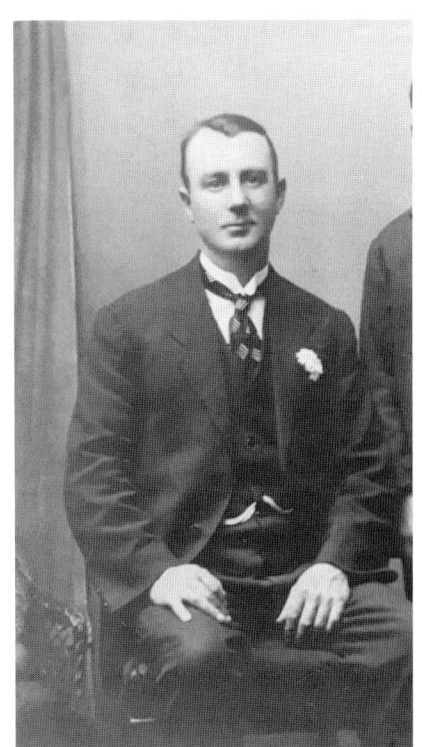

*Right*: David Parker, my great-grandfather.

*Below*: David Parker's WW1 diaries.

*Left*: Thomas John Goodwin's paperwork after being a POW.

*Below*: Thomas John Goodwin's discharge note.

*Above*: Thomas John Goodwin's certificate of service.

*Right*: Thomas John Goodwin in India.

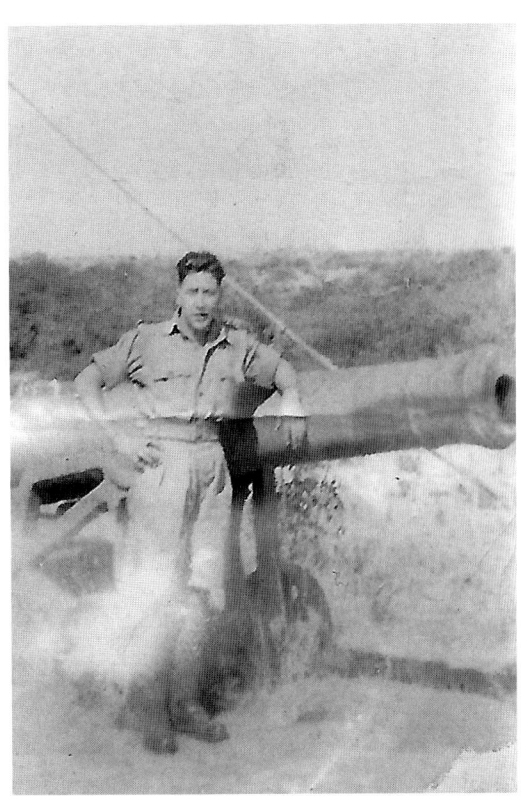

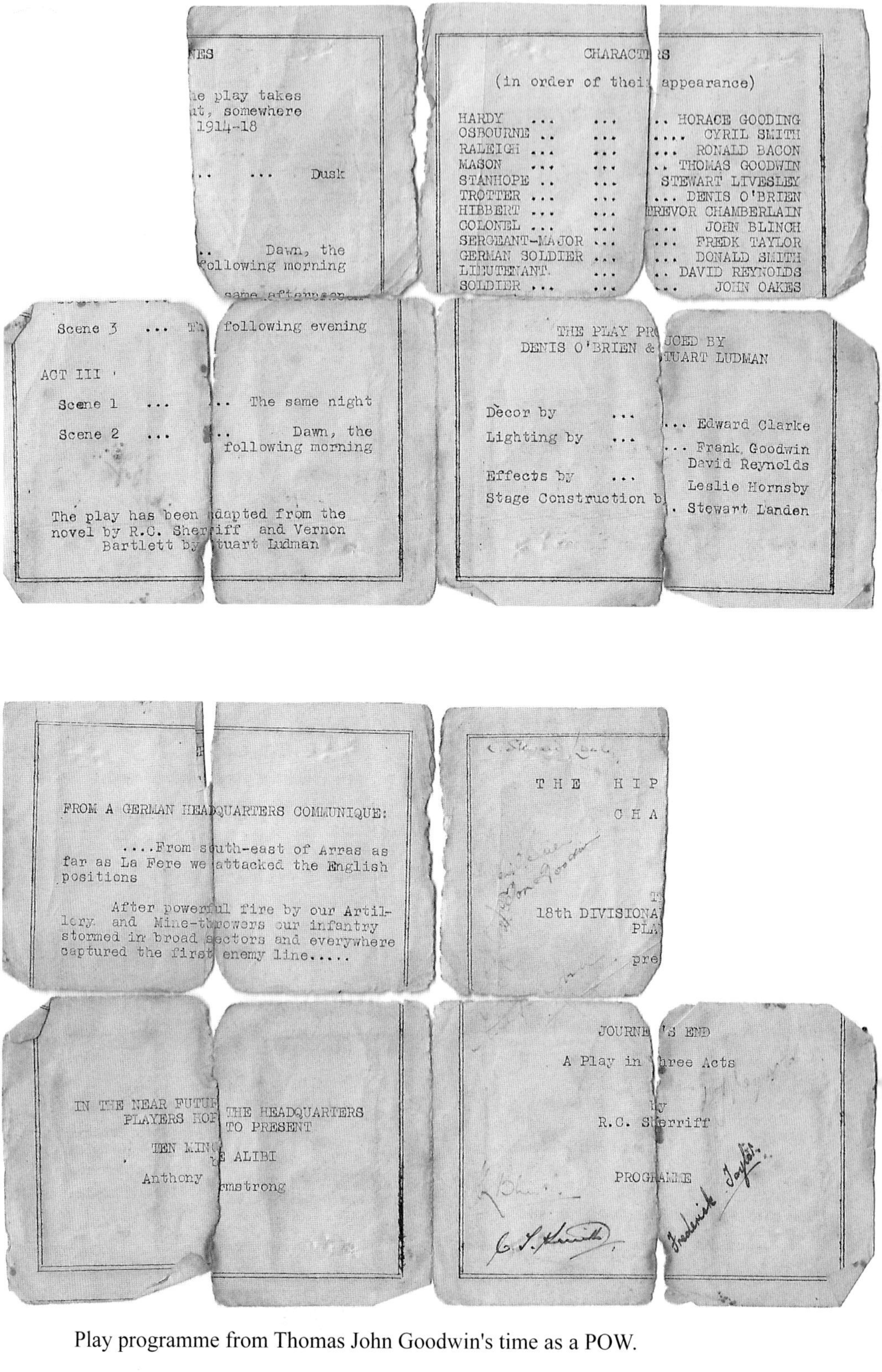

THE HIP...
CHA...

18TH DIVISIONA...
PLA...
pre...

JOURNEY'S END

A Play in Three Acts

by

R.C. Sherriff

PROGRAMME

---

FROM A GERMAN HEADQUARTERS COMMUNIQUE:

.....From south-east of Arras as far as La Fere we attacked the English positions

After powerful fire by our Artillery and Mine-throwers our infantry stormed in broad sectors and everywhere captured the first enemy line.....

IN THE NEAR FUTURE THE HEADQUARTERS
PLAYERS HOPE TO PRESENT

TEN MIN... ALIBI

Anthony ...rmstrong

---

...ES

...he play takes
...t, somewhere
...1914-18

... ... Dusk

... Dawn, the
following morning

same afternoon

Scene 3 ... ...following evening

ACT III

Scene 1 ... ... The same night
Scene 2 ... ... Dawn, the
following morning

The play has been adapted from the novel by R.C. Sherriff and Vernon Bartlett by Stuart Ludman

---

CHARACTERS

(in order of their appearance)

| HARDY | ... | ... | HORACE GOODING |
| OSBOURNE | ... | ... | CYRIL SMITH |
| RALEIGH | ... | ... | RONALD BACON |
| MASON | ... | ... | THOMAS GOODWIN |
| STANHOPE | ... | ... | STEWART LIVESLEY |
| TROTTER | ... | ... | DENIS O'BRIEN |
| HIBBERT | ... | ... | TREVOR CHAMBERLAIN |
| COLONEL | ... | ... | JOHN BLINCH |
| SERGEANT-MAJOR | ... | ... | FREDK TAYLOR |
| GERMAN SOLDIER | ... | ... | DONALD SMITH |
| LIEUTENANT | ... | ... | DAVID REYNOLDS |
| SOLDIER | ... | ... | JOHN OAKES |

THE PLAY PRODUCED BY
DENIS O'BRIEN & STUART LUDMAN

Decor by ... ... Edward Clarke
Lighting by ... ... Frank Goodwin
David Reynolds
Effects by ... Leslie Hornsby
Stage Construction by Stewart Landen

Play programme from Thomas John Goodwin's time as a POW.

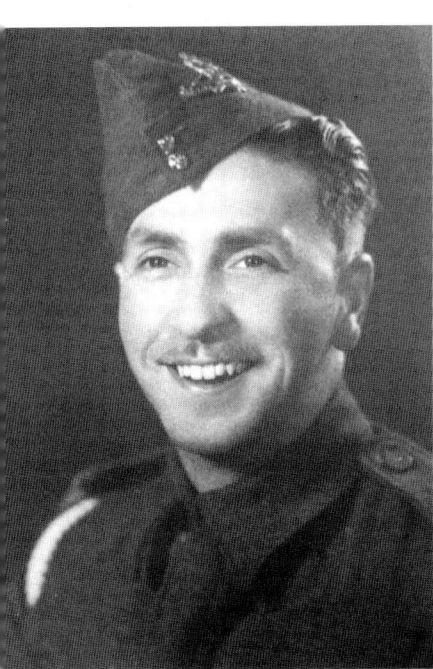

Harry Kiernan before he went to war.

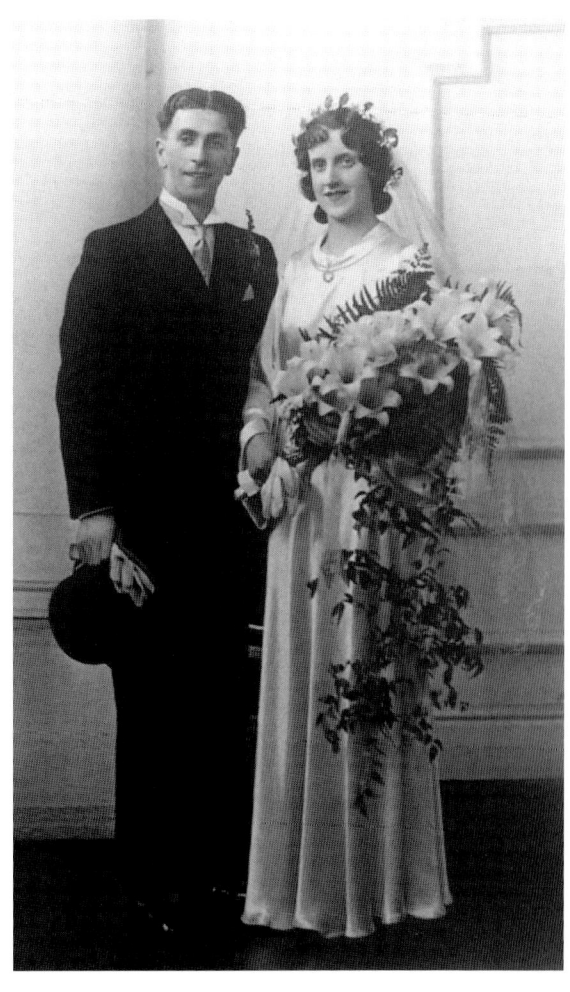

Harry Kiernan's wedding day.

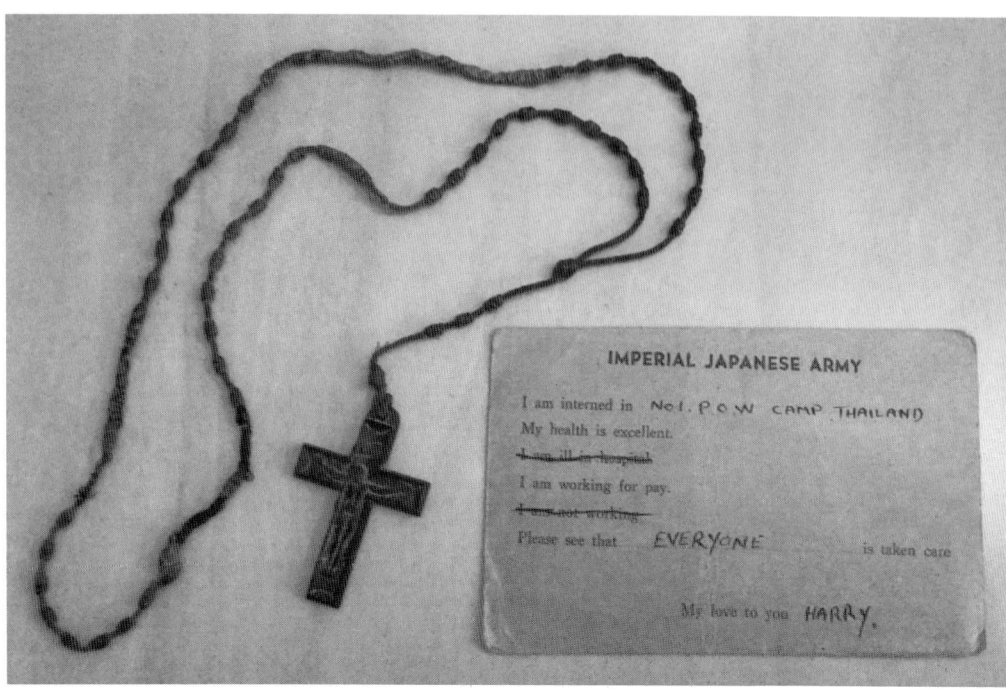

Harry Kiernan's crucifix and card that he was allowed to send home.

Kriegsgefangenenlager    Datum: 11th May, 44

My Dear Joan, how are you taking life these days. Well I hope. By the way dear excuse this card but I have explained before that letters are short. Joan are you really interested in me. I hope so. cause I could do with a friend when this trouble blows over. I hope you understand
Lots of Love John xxxx
xxxx

John Proctor, POW, letter to Joan, who would become his wife.

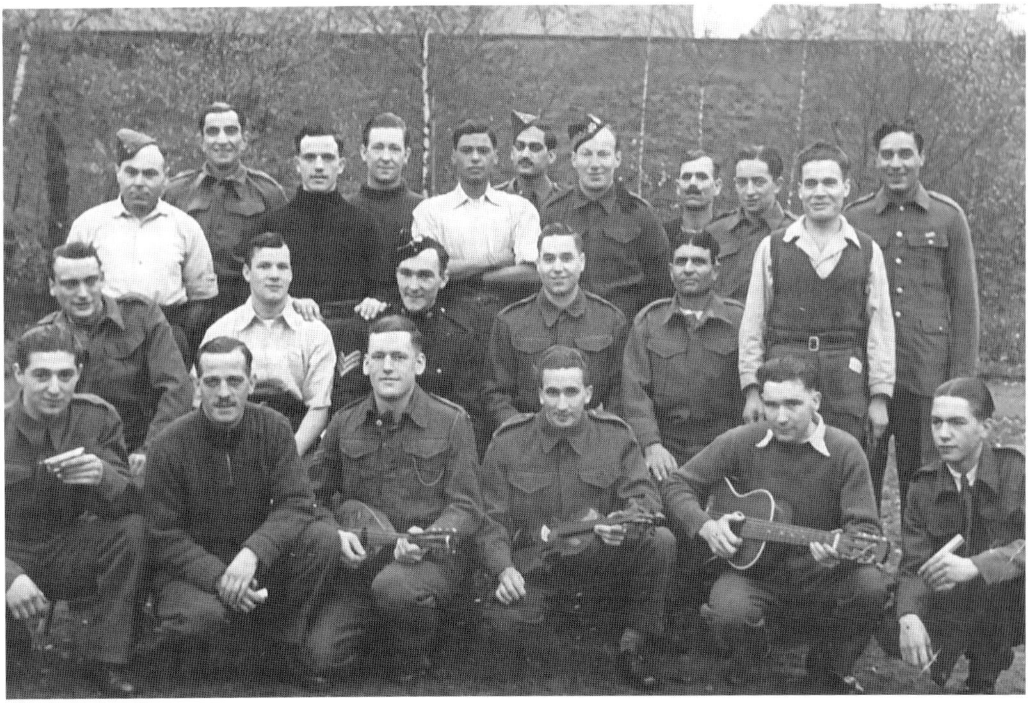

*Above*: John Proctor with a group of POWs.

*Right*: John Proctor's wedding day.

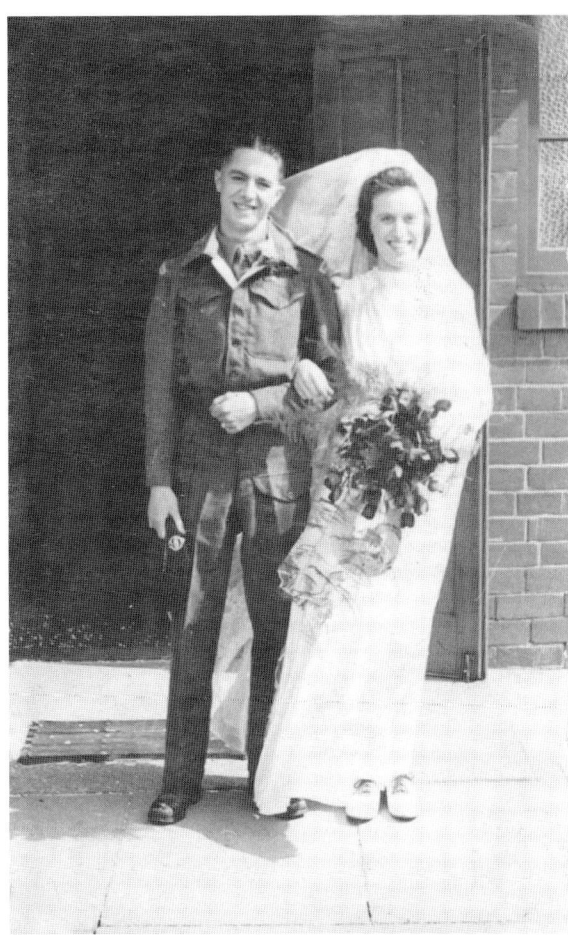

24-2-44

My Dear Joan. I have just received your letter 18/1/44. Sorry to hear about your accident I hope its not too bad. Yes my dear I wish I was home escorting you around, but don't worry I hope I shall be in a very short time. In fact I think you had better decide where we shall go on our holiday, what do you think. By the way let me have the Red Cross Leagues address. then I shall be able to convey my thanks, you understand. Is a queer do being adopted. ~~convey you the regards for the New~~ Year although a little late, but better late than never. Well dear its hard to get a letter together here; I hope you understand. Joan my dear please let me know more about yourself. By the way I hope the photos turned out good. Theres very little space left now, so Cheerio remember me to your people and don't go falling off causeways etc cause I shall want you at the station in a very short while. (I hope) Thats all for now Godbless Lots of Love
John

xxxxxx
xxxxxx

John Proctor's letter to Joan.

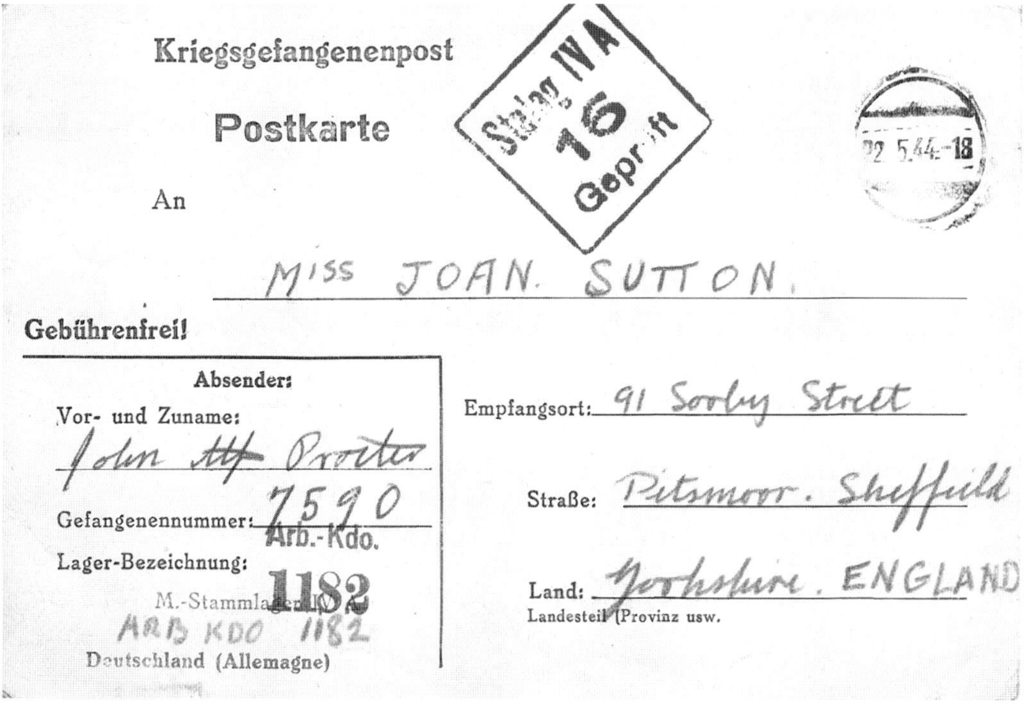
Kriegsgefangenenpost

Postkarte

Stalag IV A 16 Geprüft

22 5.44-18

An MISS JOAN. SUTTON.

Gebührenfrei!

Absender:
Vor- und Zuname: John Alf Procter
Gefangenennummer: 7590
Arb.-Kdo.
Lager-Bezeichnung: 1182
M.-Stammlager IV A
ARB KDO 1182
Deutschland (Allemagne)

Empfangsort: 91 Sorby Street
Straße: Pitsmoor. Sheffield
Land: Yorkshire. ENGLAND
Landesteil (Provinz usw.

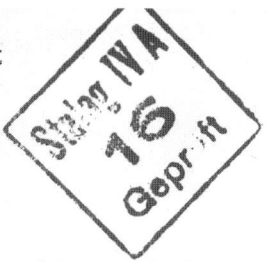

John Proctor's postcard to Joan.

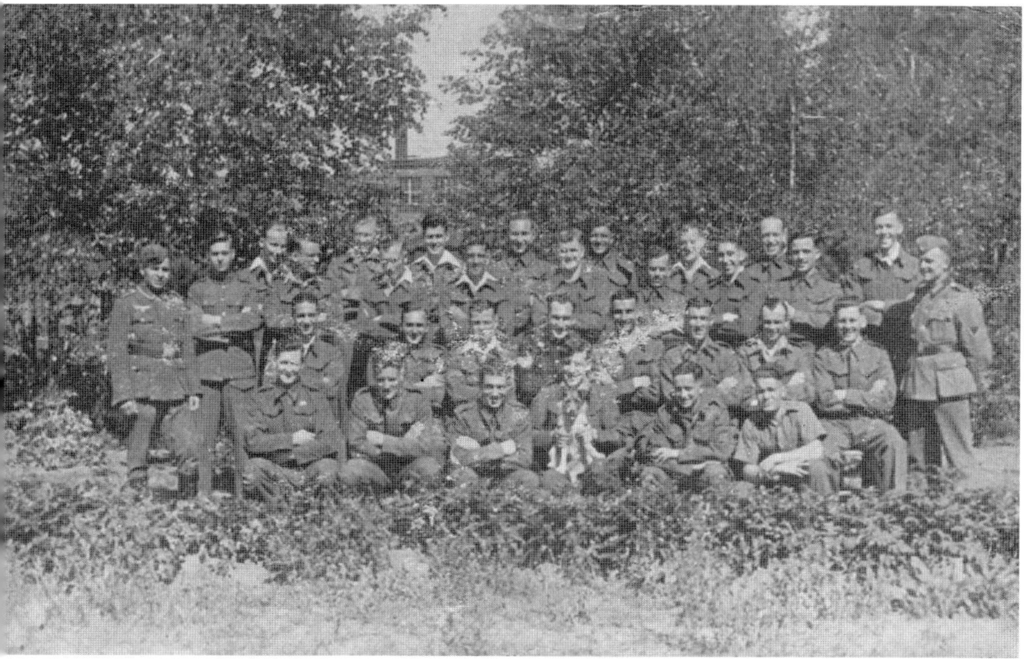

John Proctor with his squadron.

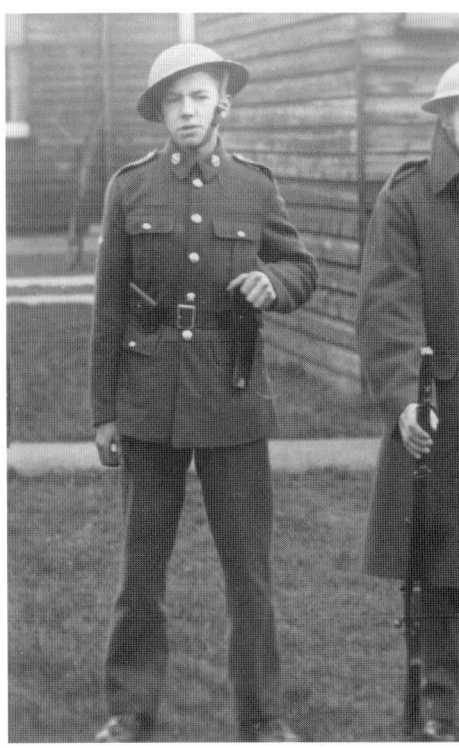

*Left*: John Proctor in uniform before going to war.

*Below*: Harry Kiernan's medals, map of the Far East and a letter confirming the war was over.

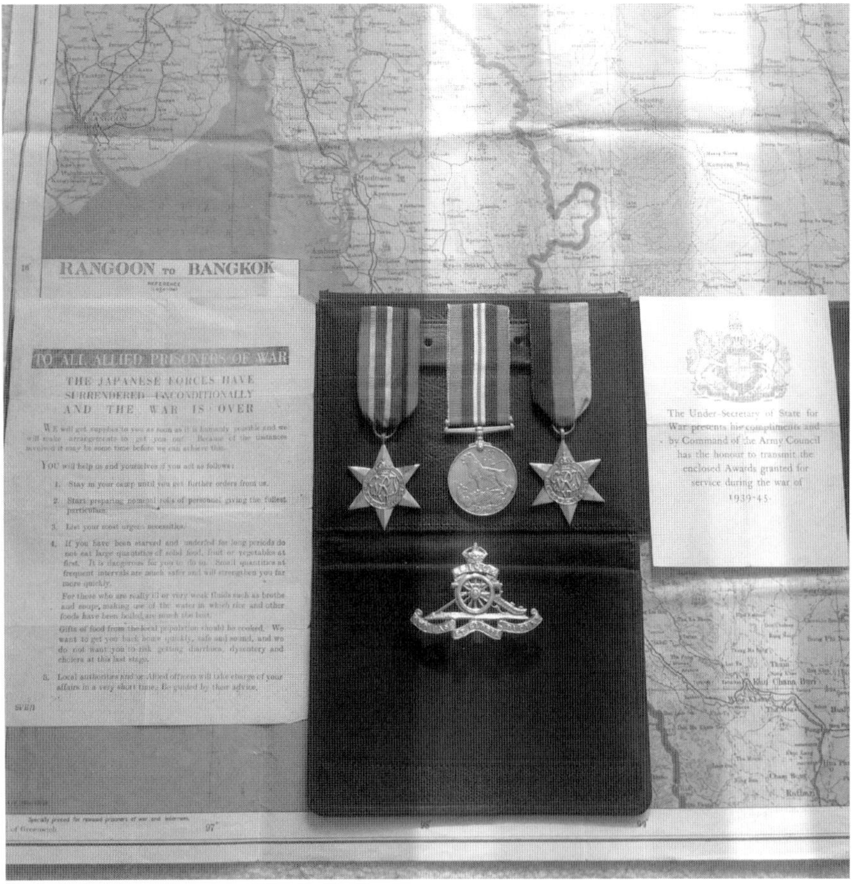

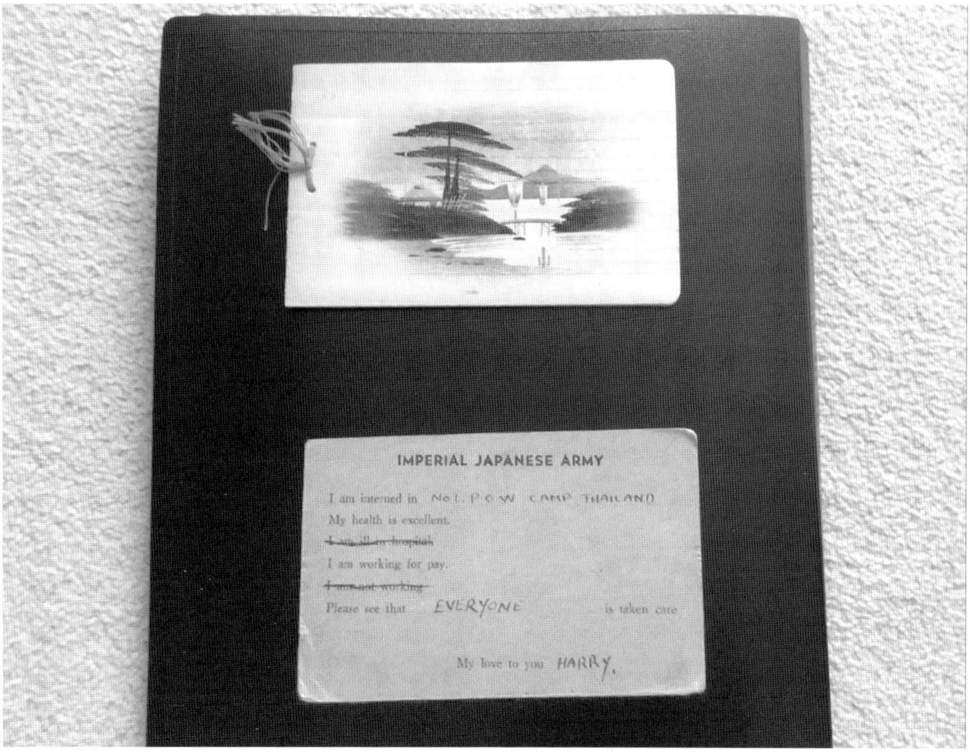


Harry Kiernan's postcard.

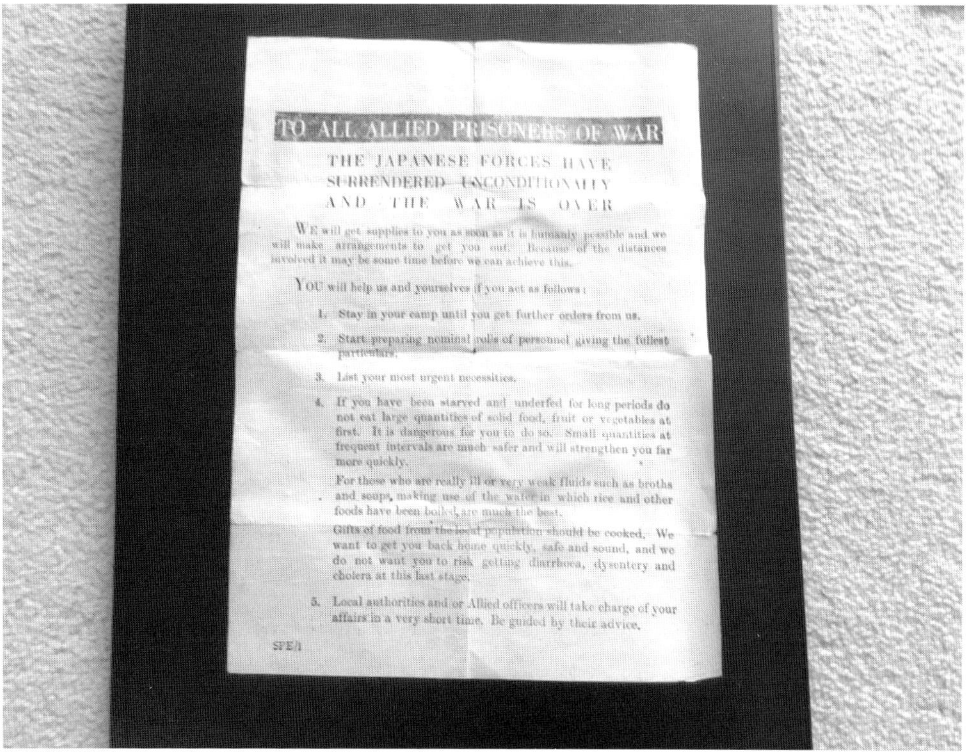

TO ALL ALLIED PRISONERS OF WAR

THE JAPANESE FORCES HAVE SURRENDERED UNCONDITIONALLY AND THE WAR IS OVER

WE will get supplies to you as soon as it is humanly possible and we will make arrangements to get you out. Because of the distances involved it may be some time before we can achieve this.

YOU will help us and yourselves if you act as follows:

1. Stay in your camp until you get further orders from us.
2. Start preparing nominal rolls of personnel giving the fullest particulars.
3. List your most urgent necessities.
4. If you have been starved and underfed for long periods do not eat large quantities of solid food, fruit or vegetables at first. It is dangerous for you to do so. Small quantities at frequent intervals are much safer and will strengthen you far more quickly.

   For those who are really ill or very weak fluids such as broths and soups, making use of the water in which rice and other foods have been boiled, are much the best.

   Gifts of food from the local population should be cooked. We want to get you back home quickly, safe and sound, and we do not want you to risk getting diarrhoea, dysentery and cholera at this last stage.
5. Local authorities and or Allied officers will take charge of your affairs in a very short time. Be guided by their advice.

SPE/1

Harry Kiernan – a letter confirming the war was over.

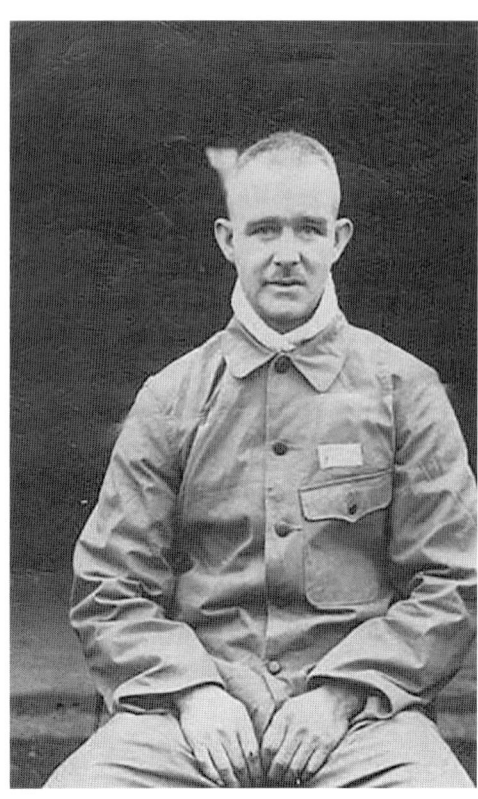

*Left*: Stanley Reader, POW and merchant seaman.

*Below*: Vivian John Clarke in a field with his comrades.

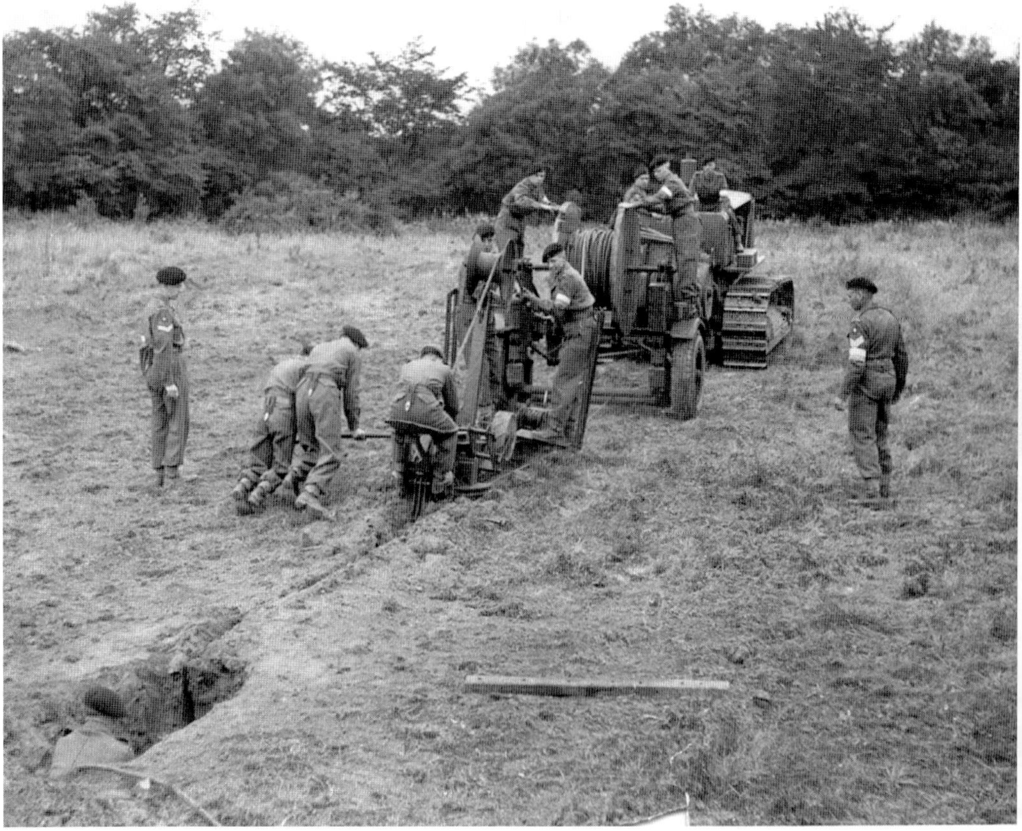

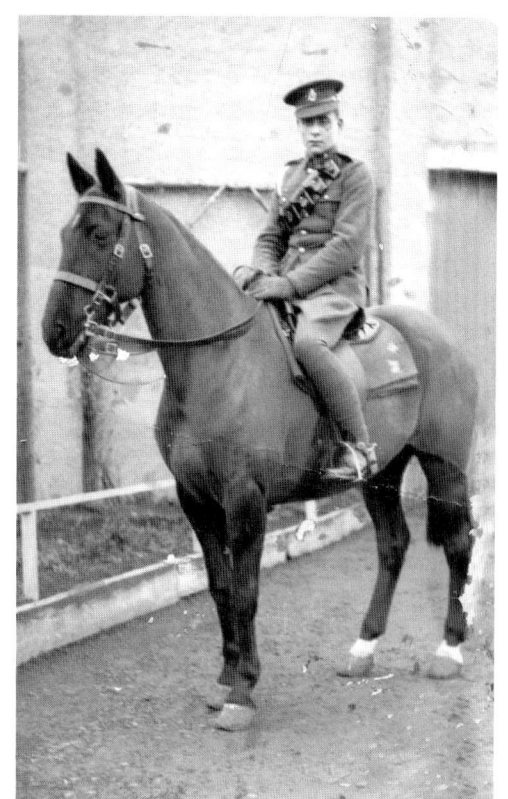

*Right*: Vivian John Clarke in uniform, mounted on a horse.

*Below*: Vivian John Clarke receiving a medal.

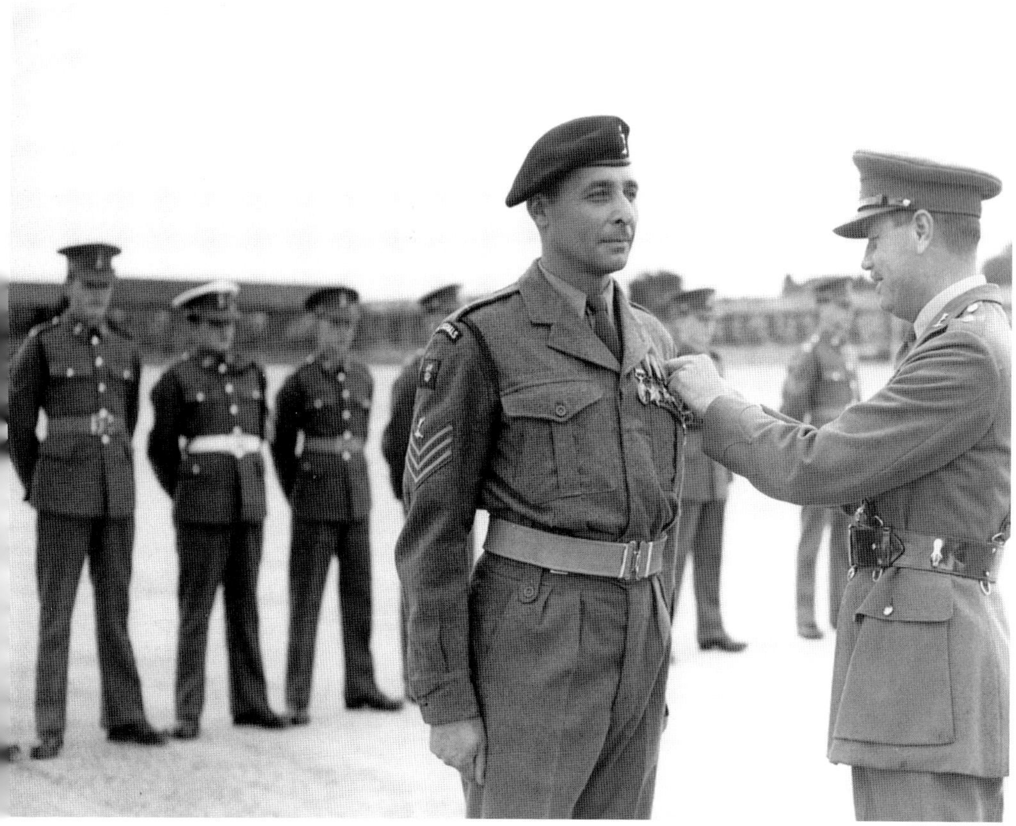

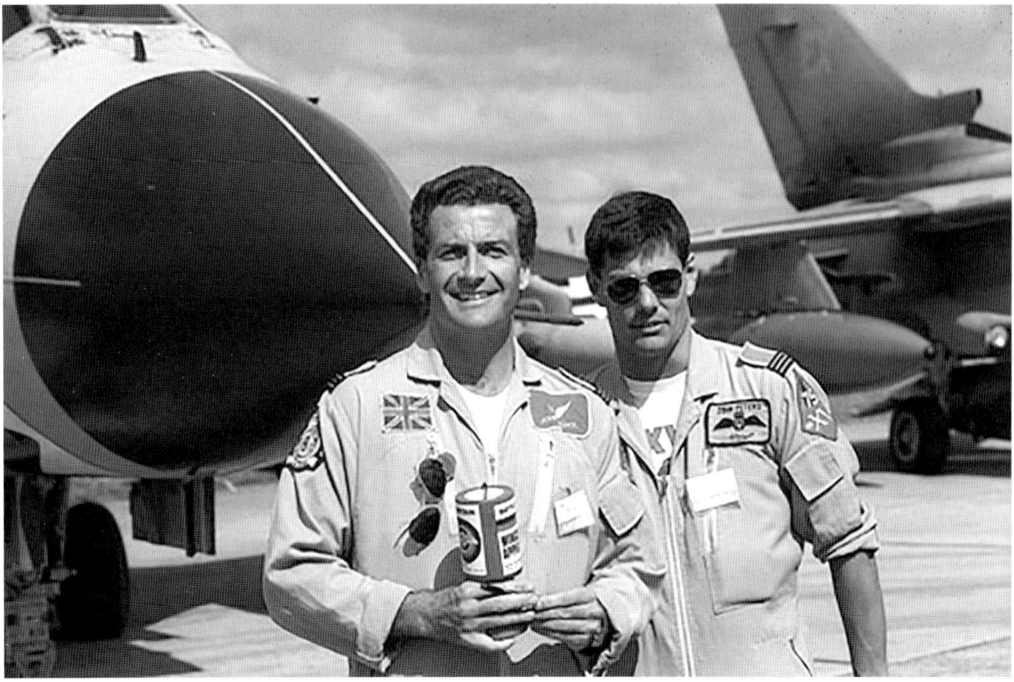

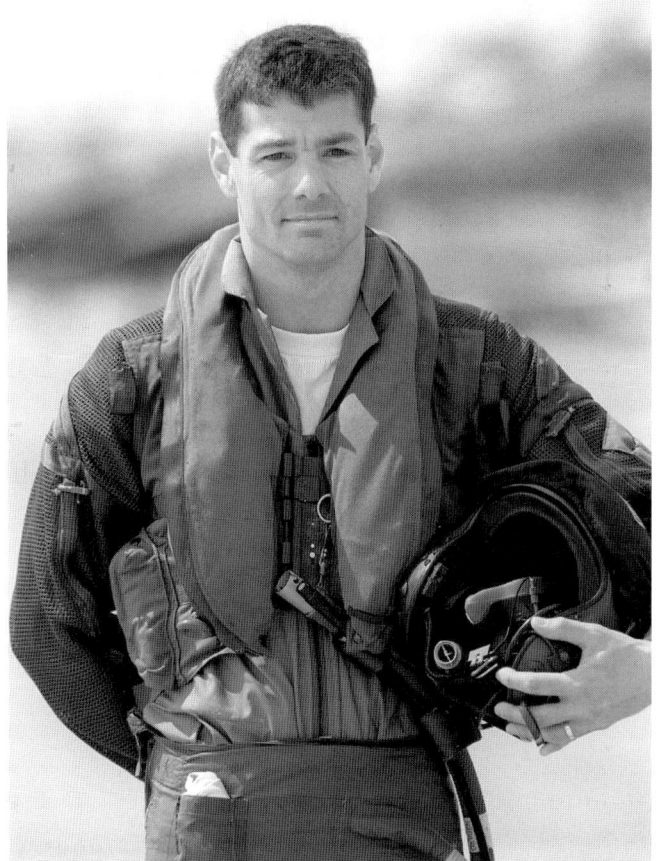

*Above*: John Peters (R) with his navigator John Nichol.

*Left*: John Peters in RAF uniform.

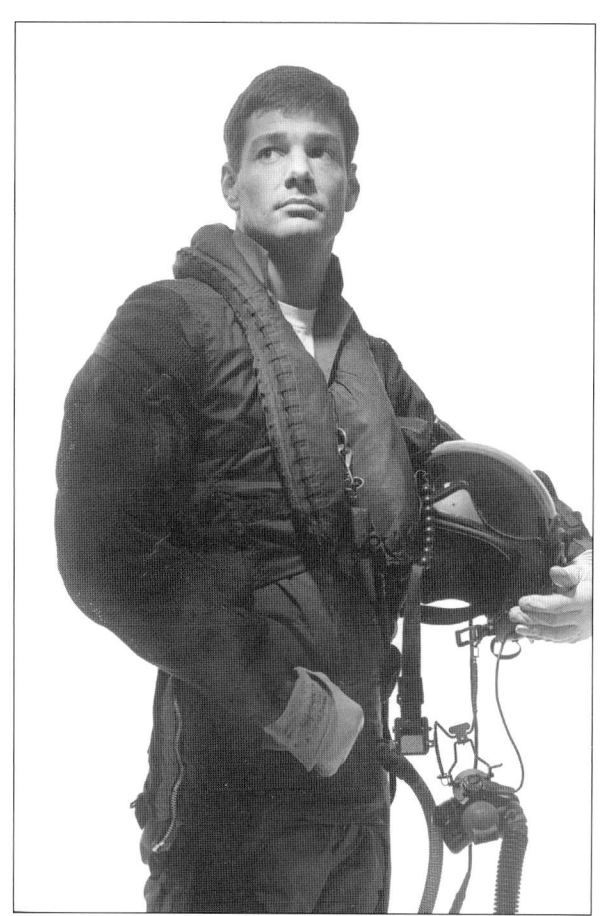

*Right*: John Peters (shoot by *FHM*).

*Below*: John now.

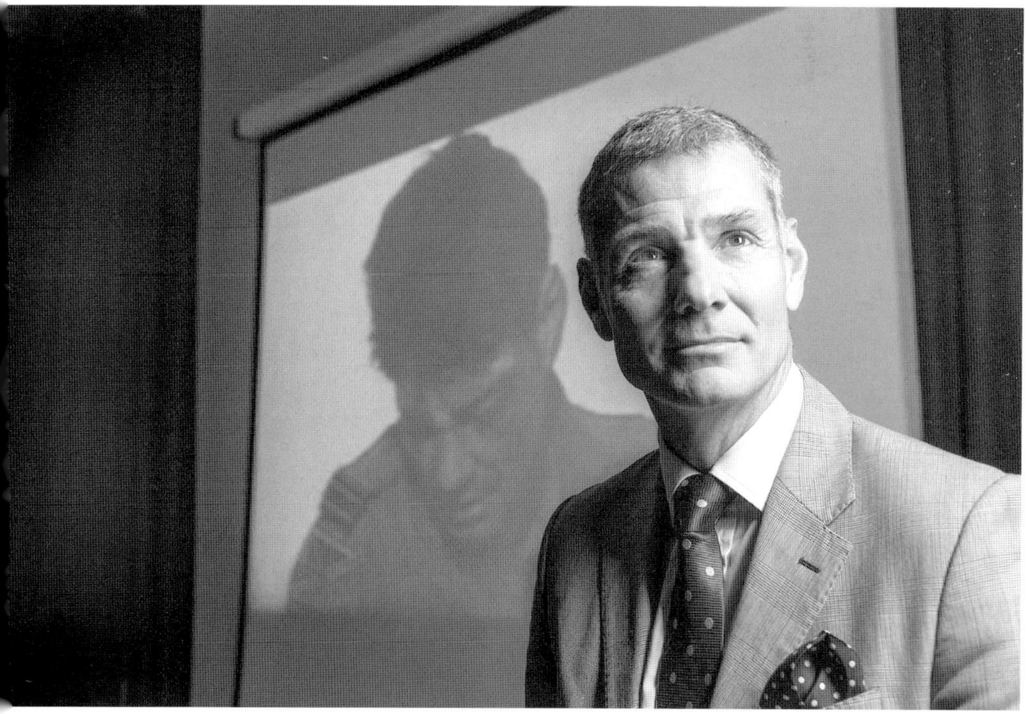

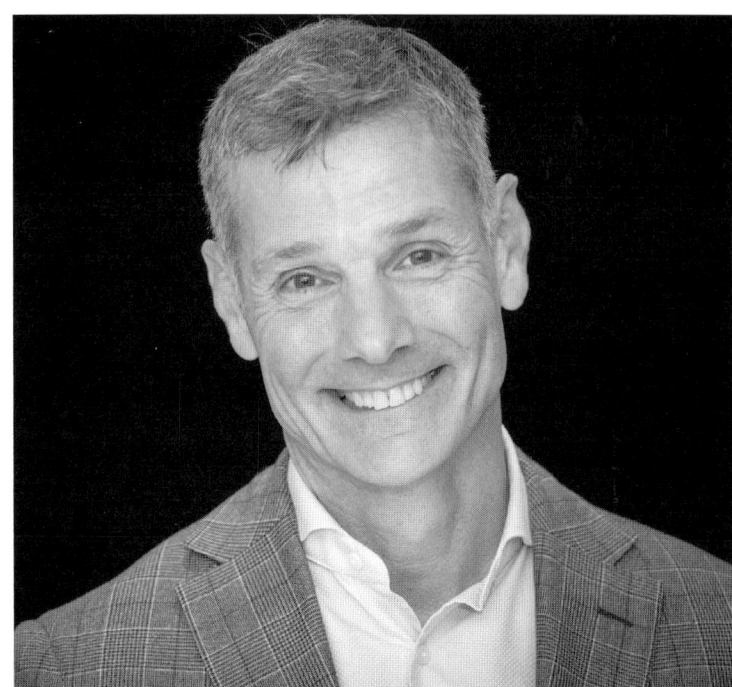

*Left*: John today.

*Below*: John in a screen grab taken from Iraqi TV during the Gulf War.

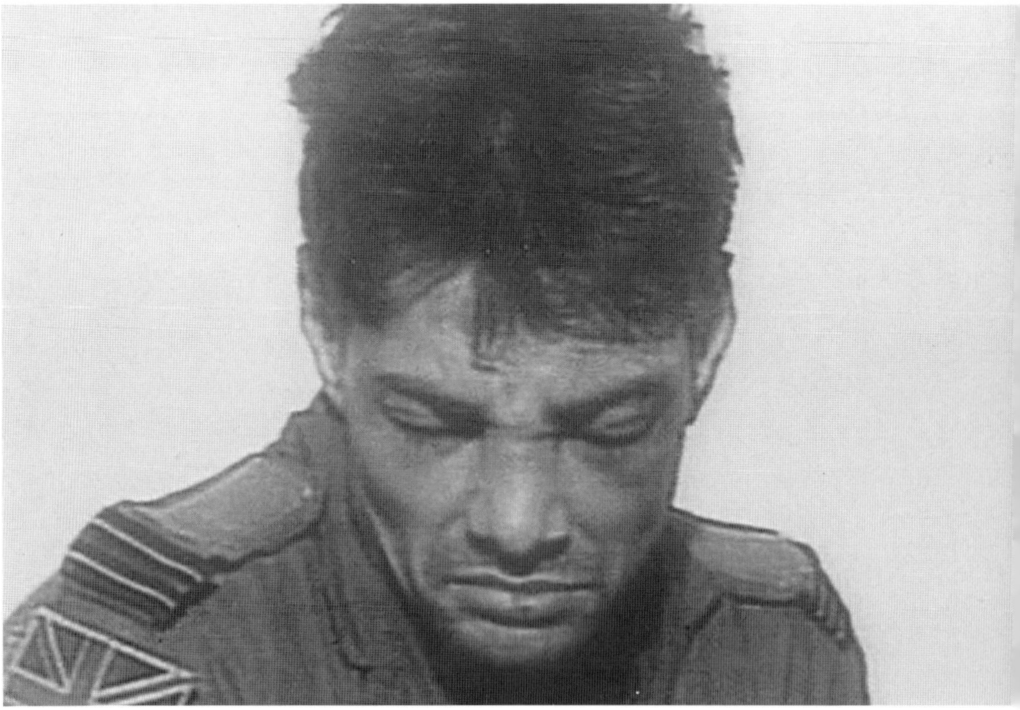

# PRISONERS OF WAR IN GERMANY – SECOND WORLD WAR

When my father came back in May 1945, he quickly met up with my mother, the woman he'd fallen in love with through letters. The inevitable happened – she became pregnant so they quickly got married just two months later in the July. I was born twelve years later in 1957. My dad was loving to me and called me 'Bubble'.

But there was a very dark side too. Dad liked to go out for a drink at weekends and didn't like it if Mum wouldn't go out with him too. One of my very first memories, when I was aged around 3, is of living in the countryside where there were a few odd country pubs. Dad wanted to go to a pub and Mum had said no. He then went out and came home worse for wear. She had this little TV and he came in and just walked over and cut the plug so she couldn't watch it anymore. Then a full-scale argument broke out. I ran away and remembered sitting on the stairs with my brother looking after me as pots and pans were flying out of the kitchen.

Another memory was of my dad putting his hands around my mum's neck. But we never knew or understood what triggered it. But as I got older, I began to hear snippets of what it was like for him as a prisoner of war. His health was never good. I remember he'd wake having nightmares. My mother explained that right up to me being born, Dad had been taken to various hospitals for shock treatments and was on medication a lot for his mental health. He couldn't keep certain jobs down.

One problem was that he could not stand being indoors. He had to be outside, so he found work on the road as a lorry driver. He delivered the *Sheffield Star* newspaper.

But although he tried his best, his mental health plagued him. At one point doctors even planned to do a lobotomy on him but he panicked and begged my mother to sign the papers to get him out of the hospital before they could operate. Other times Dad had been put in padded cells in hospital because he'd been trying to harm himself. He never hit me. But it did lead to problems at home. He shouted a lot and New Year's Eve was the worst time. He'd drink too much and then I'd see arguments that were not pleasant. I was always nervy, always thinking: is he about to go off on one? Nonetheless I did feel loved. I knew he loved me and my mother.

And as the years passed, I learnt more about his time as a prisoner of war which helped explain his behaviour. The camp he'd been held in was near Dresden. After the Allies bombed the city, the Germans used the prisoners of war to go into the city to clear up and check for bodies.

Dad said that the sights he saw never left him. He saw people burnt, stuck to the roads, dissolved. He told us of how he'd go into the cellars of buildings to check for people. The civilians had thought they'd be safe there but Dad found many of them dead, sitting as they had been hours earlier, holding their babies or playing cards. The blasts of the bombs had sucked all the air out of the cellars and they had suffocated.

Dad had been hit in the head by a rifle but he'd also witnessed other prisoners, friends, getting shot.

Another time he told of how he and a fellow prisoner wanted to go the toilet and the latrines were outside of the huts. To get to the latrines they'd have to come out with their hands up because there were guards all the way around. Dad explained that the guards nodded to let the prisoners come out and use the latrine but as he and his friend were walking out with their hands up one of the guards shot the man next to him through the head. No warning. Just for sport. They were Bulgarian guards, Dad told us. 'They were worse than the Germans,' he used to say quietly.

I tried to understand all he had been through. He had clearly had such terrible times. But we always were on eggshells, thinking: why does he have to make life hell? I'd go to friends houses whose parents were not like Dad and I would think: why isn't it like this at our house? You'd never know what mood Dad would be in. We couldn't get inside his head. But in so many ways he was a good father. He wasn't a big built man and was always thin but he was strong. He wasn't a shirker either and worked hard. He loved anything where he could use his hands or anything mechanical. He had more strength in his arms than a lot of bigger men.

But he had to be outdoors. He couldn't stand being confined. As I got older I understood why – he had been in solitary confinement for trying to escape. It made sense. Mum explained to me that in the early years after his release, Dad's health suffered and he couldn't digest very much. He had only weighed four-and-a-half stone when he'd got back to Britain. I know Japanese prisoners got it very hard but depending on which camp prisoners were in in Germany, it could be as cruel.

Mum explained to me that he'd been on starvation rations and had survived on just black bread and potato. The prisoners would catch hedgehogs and cook them encased in clay. Dad had told her that when you took the clay off, it peeled everything back so there was never much meat left on the hedgehog. But anything to survive.

Even as I got older, I could tell Dad's nightmares never went away. As they aged, they had to sleep in separate rooms as he would lash out in his sleep. The worst time each year was Valentine's Day because that was the time of year when Dresden was bombed over three nights. I dreaded that time of year. In time I left home and had my own children. I don't know if the years mellowed him but my dad opened up more to two of my three sons. He still only came out with snippets but he wrote down certain things I didn't understand. On one little page Dad wrote:

*March to Luxemburg.*
*Train cattle trucks to Poland. Various work. (They were in the mines)*
*Then buildings were down. Winter of 40/41 very very cold.*
*Got billeted in a large mansions had been a wonderful place. Experienced frostbite to hands and was in hospital doctor put a brick with my hand prints in it in a glass case.*

He jotted things like this but that I never understood what they meant.

In 1994 Dad had open heart surgery. Then in the year 2000 there was an article in the local paper. It was about a lady who had found a Bible and in it it said it belonged to J. Procter. I read the piece and took it to my dad. He had a read and said: 'That's my Bible.' It turned out he'd had it during his time as a prisoner of war which had been given to him by the Red Cross. In it, he had written: *Should anything happen to me, please give this to my mother.*

We contacted the lady who sent him the Bible. A few weeks later Dad went to visit her to thank her. I found it strange as Dad had always said he was an atheist after all he'd been through. Yet, seeing him take the time to get this Bible, and to keep it and treasure it, shows it must have been of some comfort to him. Dad was a member of the National Prisoner of War Association and he was referred to Combat Stress for counselling.

The first time he went, he found it very hard to open up to people about what he'd seen. He'd be talking, but sitting in a chair and gripping the arms of the chair so tight that his knuckles went white.

He went for two weeks at a time twice a year and we noticed that he began to open up more. They did a wonderful job with him. It was fifty years later than his return, but it did restore some normality.

Eventually my mother got Alzheimer's and was taken into a care home. Around this point, and perhaps thanks to the counselling, Dad used to say: 'I so regret how I was.'

I think he wished he could turn back the clock.

In 2007 Dad died. He'd had his last Combat Stress counselling sessions just seven months before he passed away. He'd had various strokes and had been in hospital. I was at his side when he died.

That year, I went to clean out things. As I looked, I found some paperwork. It was Dad's medical records. I never knew it but he had sent away for them and had kept them.

I sat down and read them. And as I did, it dawned on me: This is why he was the way was.

I saw that although Dad had had many psychiatric problems as a result of being a prisoner of war, he got no help at all except for going to the GP for tablets. There was no early counselling offered or support of any kind. He was simply expected to come home, get a job and carry on. It was true of so many of that era. There was no help. Prisoners of war went to get their tablets from the doctor and that was that. Alcohol was a big problem for many ex-POWs and made things so much worse.

Knowing what I know now, after reading his medical records, I can see why he was so damaged. I just wish I'd have sat with him more. Some days he didn't want to open up and other days he did but life's always busy.

I should have sat down and said: 'Go on, Dad, then, tell us.'

Many children of prisoners of war say that they wished they'd asked their fathers more and yet felt awkward and often wanted their father to start the conversation first, to ensure he would be comfortable with talking. The difficulty was that it was often impossible to tell when that man might feel comfortable and when he simply wanted to shut down. The study by Jeffrey and Bradford concluded that many of the prisoners of war in their care actually displayed psychopath tendencies when compared to other patients with anxiety and they wrote:

> the POW patient cannot on his own initiative continue a prolonged train of activity, and to read a book makes him fall asleep. He seems to be in need of re-education, but can his curiosity be re-awakened or can sufficiently attractive goals be presented? Will the return to civilian life be sufficiently stimulating to the reintegration of his mental or intellectual life?[25]

The study makes for fascinating, if not a little despairing, reading. The resounding summary seems to be that if a man is damaged from being a prisoner of war, there is little that can be done. Yet so many men seemed to manage. Many did find work again and did return to a relationship with their wives, even having more children.

So what was it that made some men crumble from being a prisoner of war and some men seem to thrive?

# Chapter Five

# Japan and the Far East

'Dad said whatever you do, don't buy creosote. "Back on the railway I had to paint the sleepers with creosote," he said. "And we'd stand there naked and get creosote on your body that would burn like hell."'

Kevin Goodwin, on his father Thomas Goodwin,
POW in the Far East

'[At] the 55 Kilometre Camp at Kohn Kuhn, Burma, were collected the majority of the casualties of the railway in Burma in the second half of 1943, that is 1,800 patients, of whom 500 suffered from ulcer of the leg. There was an odd ulcer of the hand, back, forearm or thigh but the vast majority had one or more ulcers on the lower extremity, usually in the distal half.'

'Surgery in Japanese Prison Camps', Coates, A. E. Anz Journal of Surgery, Volume 15, 1946, p.151

No one believed Singapore would fall. That was the general consensus. The naval base at Singapore – the Gibraltar of the Far East – was where the British fleet was kept during the Second World War in case of any threat of aggression. Nevertheless, as war dragged on, more and more British troops were sent to defend Malaya and Singapore as the Japanese advanced. Soon there were 85,000 British troops on the

## JAPAN AND THE FAR EAST

Singapore island commanded by Lieutenant General Arthur Percival. Although 30,000 Japanese men had advanced down the Malayan Peninsular, the British believed Singapore would not fall. First, there was impregnable jungle to pass through. Second, the island had 85,000 British troops. Third, and perhaps most damaging of all, was British colonial arrogance that no force could possibly defeat theirs.

When the Japanese did strike, they took Percival by surprise. They bombed the RAF base meaning Allied pilots could not defend the skies. And as for their land soldiers, they did not take prisoners. Literally. Japanese soldiers were renowned for their ruthless brutality. They pushed through Singapore at such speed the British could not react either in time or effectively. Two Navy ships – the *Prince of Wales* and *Repulse* – were sent to defend Singapore but were sunk by the Japanese.

Singapore fell. General Percival surrendered – something the Japanese with their culture of never surrendering could never respect or understand. Winston Churchill would later call the fall of Singapore 'the worst disaster and largest capitulation in British history', not least because the invading army was half Britain's size. After conquering Singapore, the Japanese took 100,000 British and commonwealth prisoners. If those prisoners had believed that their incarceration might be similar to that of their European counterparts in Germany, they were sadly mistaken. Germany had signed up to the Geneva Convention. Japan had reluctantly signed but not formalised this in their parliament. Reiterating the Japanese cultural belief that surrender is the greatest shame is important and reflects their ill-treatment of prisoners as a result: they could never respect or understand a man who had not fought to the death.

The prisoners were transported through hot, humid and incredibly uncomfortable conditions to camps such as Changi in Singapore and Tamajao 241 in Thailand. In a telegram, the Japanese government had agreed to adhere to the Geneva Convention in the treatment of English, Australian, Canadian, New Zealand and Indian prisoners of war. However, this would prove to be a lie. Not only did the Japanese consider the prisoners dishonourable and not worthy of respect for being taken prisoner, but they also administered corporal punishment among their own ranks in the army and so, brutality was the norm.

Prisoners were transported to their camps in 'hell ships'. These ships would be the prisoners' first taste of how the Japanese would treat them. Cramped in overcrowded, packed cargo holds in the ships with little air, no food and barely any water, some prisoners died of dysentery, suffocation or dehydration before they even reached the camp. Other prisoners died when Allied planes bombed the ships, not knowing they contained British or Commonwealth soldiers. For those that did survive the voyage, they were often delirious with the heat and dehydration by the time they reached their camp.

Those who were kept at Changi prison in Singapore were forced into labour to build an air strip for the Japanese air force. News of treatment in Changi reached home to British newspapers. At first, it was heavily sanitised. In one report in the *Daily Record* soon after Singapore fell, Lieutenant General Percival told reporters 'We have enough to eat and our daily needs are satisfied but we should like a little more water.'[1]

But of course, treatment would get worse. Japanese camps were the harshest in any theatre of war. Most prisoners were put on a starvation diet of just one small bowl of rice at the end of each day. The Red Cross tried to send parcels but many were retained by the Japanese guards and never reached their recipients. In many men this soon led to a vitamin B-1 deficiency called beriberi disease. The word beriberi was a Singhalese word meaning 'I can't, I can't' or 'extreme weakness', and was caused by the lack of thiamine in the prisoners' diets. Beriberi led to muscle atrophy, heart and nerve damage and even death. Coupled with the forced labour Japanese camps enforced upon the prisoners, many men died of exhaustion or malnutrition.

Punishments were also harsh. Face-slapping was common and an almost daily occurrence for prisoners and could be dished out for something as innocuous as forgetting to salute a guard. Other punishments were more inventive and involved holding a heavy stone above the man's head for hours (being beaten if he dropped it) and being placed in a confined space for many hours in the heat of the day. Other examples include men being forced to sit or kneel on fast-growing bamboo for days until it grew into their body, causing blood loss and gangrene.

Prisoners often did not receive letters and so could not write home. Many died of the work, the heat, beriberi or being executed at the whim of a guard.

In fact, many news reports in 1942, featured letters which had reached home many weeks later in which inmates expressed that they were being treated well. One letter included: 'The prisoners of war are now in Changi barracks, east of the island. Food is plentiful and of European standard and the water supply is good.'[2]

The reality was of course far, far different. Not only were British and Commonwealth prisoners of war being beaten, tortured and starved, in some cases Japanese guards were actually resorting to cannibalism – eating prisoners of war.[3] Other prisoners were blindfolded, made to sit cross-legged and be used as training for target practise for Japanese soldiers. Those who were not shot successfully were bayoneted to death.

It was in the interest of the government and Ministry of Defence to keep these atrocities from the British public, for fear of destroying morale. But some news did creep home.

One report published in a newspaper featured alleged spying in a camp. After an investigation into 'spying' in the prison, British prisoners of war faced even harsher treatment:

> Conditions under which internees were detained were rigorous in the extreme. From eight o'clock in the morning until ten at night they had to sit up straight on the bare floor with their knees up, and were not allowed to relax, or to put their hands on the floor, or to talk or to

move except to go to the lavatory. Any infraction involved a beating by the guards. Nearly all the inmates suffered from enteritis or dysentery. No soap, towel, toilet articles or handkerchief were permitted.[4]

Another story which shocked British readers was the treatment of women and children civilians who were also held prisoner in Changi.

> Three women taken from Changi prison were detained in exactly the same conditions as the men, and shared cells with male prisoners of all races. They were afforded no privacy and any attempt on the part of the European men to screen them was broken down by the guards. They were subjected to insults and obscene gestures by Japanese prisoners who, with the assent of the guards, tried to compel them to perform the most sordid tasks.[5]

One civilian lady who was imprisoned in Changi was Lady Thomas, wife of Sir Shenton Thomas, Governor of the Straits Settlements in Singapore. She said: 'It was dreadful to see men who had been taken away big and burly coming back weighing only five stone.'

The bread ration in Changi was a piece four inches square and half an inch wide and this was for two men for twenty-four hours. But the real hell was for the men who were forced to work on the Burma Railway – or Death Railway as it would later be known. In 1942, the Japanese began using their Allied prisoners of war to work on a railway that would link Thailand and Burma. This railway would be 415km long and would also need over 600 bridges including viaducts. The Japanese forces built around 100 camps along the planned railway where prisoners of war would be held during the labour.

The work involved first clearing large areas of dense jungle – backbreaking physical work. Food was usually one bowl of rice at the end of each day and soldiers were forced to work in blistering tropical heat, often wearing only a rag around their loins. The Japanese wanted the railway built as quickly as possible and dished out cruel punishments to anyone who did not work at the speed required, including beatings, lashings, forced solitary confinement, withdrawal of food and water and even execution. It is now believed that 13,000 Allied prisoners of war died building the Death Railway. Most died of disease – cholera, malaria, dysentery and tropical ulcers – while many were executed or beaten to death.

For medics and doctors held prisoner, they did their best to help their ailing fellow soldiers but often didn't have the equipment they needed. One doctor wrote of how he had to perform surgery on fellow prisoners but that 'no electric bulbs or batteries were allowed by the Japanese'. Incredibly, the doctor was able to operate on a soldier who had rectal ulcers: 'Proctoscopes were fashioned out of tin and an instrument three inches long, one inch in diameter with slightly inbent edges, transmitted sunlight reflected from a mirror for several inches up the rectum.'[6]

Many doctors wrote afterwards of the sense of impotence at wanting to treat their fellow soldiers but simply not having the tools needed to do so.

Dr A.E. Coates also wrote of his time in Japanese camps:

> By June, 1943, conditions among prisoners of war on the Burma-Siam railway were deplorable. Sick and injured were kept in their working camps for months and when sufficient number were collected or the camp moved on, the abandoned huts would be used to house the patients. Such a so-called hospital was the 55 Kilometre Camp at Kohn Kuhn, Burma. There were collected the majority of the casualties of the railway in Burma in the second half of 1943, that is 1800 patients, of whom 500 suffered from ulcer of the leg. There was an odd ulcer of the hand, back, forearm or thigh but the vast majority had one or more ulcers on the lower extremity, usually in the distal half.[7]

## THE TRAUMA OF CAPTIVITY

This doctor had to perform 114 lower-limb amputations in the camps for ulcers destroying the lower leg and foot. The anaesthetic he used was cocaine given spinally and the antiseptic used was alcohol which they made from rice. He wrote that immersing his hands in this alcohol before performing operations was successful and none of his surgeries resulted in infection from his hands. He wrote:

> The wards were bamboo huts provided with wooden platforms on each side of a central passage. The patients lay on the platforms. No beds were available until 1945, when the Japanese ordered all improvised beds, of which there were a few possessed by officers, to be put into the acute surgical ward. Bugs were a pest, and after a lot of persuasion the Japanese allowed the wooden floors to be pulled up every week for cleaning.[8]

The writings from men – doctors, soldiers, officers – all make for harrowing reading and of unthinkable conditions and cruelty. But when VJ (Victory over Japan) Day came on 2 September, 1945, the prisoners of war now faced another tumultuous change: coming home.

Jack Clarke was a prisoner of war in the Far East for four years and worked on the Burma Railway. His son Dave Clarke was born in 1948 just after his father returned. His father didn't talk a lot about his experience but was angry and bitter that his time there was not recognised. He never lived to see compensation.

### 'Dad was still having nightmares in the late sixties'

Dave Clarke, son of Jack Clarke, POW on the Burma Railway

My dad's name was Jack Clarke. He was a big man at around 6ft 2in, he weighed 14 stone and used to box in the army before the war. I was age 10 when I knew he was a POW. I would only be about 8

## JAPAN AND THE FAR EAST

when we used to drive to see the fellow ex-prisoner, so I think I had an idea from 8 years old. But he'd only talk about it occasionally.

I learnt that during Dad's time in the camps he suffered from the usual diseases such as beriberi and malaria. He also had huge scars on the backs of his legs which were from jungle ulcers. The only treatment for them was to hold a man down and clean the ulcer out with a razor blade and take flesh out and try to clean it – an extremely painful process. Dad and all his comrades had jungle ulcers. Dad also had scars all over his back. When I asked about them he said they were from being beaten by a Japanese guard. He was also scarred from working on the Burma Railway known as the Death Railway. He'd been digging stones to go under the railway sleepers and he fell down the slope and because they worked virtually naked he tore all the skin off his back. He also told me about his scars on his back – if you didn't salute the Japanese or Korean guards quickly enough they'd beat you badly.

The punishments were equally harsh. One Christmas he spent Christmas Eve standing up holding a heavy log and every time he dropped it, he'd get a whack. Finally at the end of the war, Dad was shipped slowly back to Rangoon and placed in a hospital there for a few months so they could help them put some weight back on. Dad had started at 14 stone. When he'd left the camp he was only seven stone. When he finally arrived back in the UK, war in Europe had been over for almost a year and most people in Britain had no knowledge of the Far East war. There were also still rationing. Because he was an ex-prisoner he got extra rations but one time there was a lady in a shop who berated him, saying: 'What's a bloke like you doing with extra rations?' It upset him. He needed them to regain his strength.

When Dad came back he was very restless. He left the army and joined the police, then left the police and rejoined the army. Given his background, the army was the only family he ever knew. Dad had been born in 1917 and his father had died in the First World War of wounds before he was born. His mother remarried almost immediately. And his mother then had eight children but he was given up because we think her second husband told her to get rid of him because he wasn't his. So, Dad was abandoned by his mother. He then spent the next few years being shunted to two maiden aunts in Wolverhampton. They were of the Victorian school of child upbringing and very strict so he left to join the army underage as soon as could. After all, his mother didn't want him and he had no father and the army was the only real family he ever knew.

That led to an inability to make friends, compounded by being a prisoner because the friends he did have, some of them died. Dad married my mother in 1947. Then I was born in 1948. He had a bit of a temper. He never hit us but could explode at the drop of a hat. He was fit but always had underlying health conditions because of what he'd gone through, one of them being permanent stomach problems. In the 1970s, all the ex-POWs were called up and tested by the University of Liverpool Tropical Diseases Unit and hundreds of ex-POWs from the Far East were found to be carrying tape worm, Dad too. So that explained the constantly upset stomach.

As I got older I tried to get Dad to talk. He'd talk about having to hold up the log for hours, or the scars on his back. He'd tell me that the worst guards were the Korean guards, actually worse than the Japanese. He explained it was because Japan occupied Korea in the thirties and they conscripted lots of Koreans into the Japanese military and they were very cruel. He said the only decent Japanese guard he ever met was a Christian. So, you'd get odd snippets about what had happened. But he was part of a generation that didn't really talk about it. During a lot of my childhood Dad was in the army and was until 1962. He's got a long service good conduct medal.

I went to seventeen different schools and moved around a lot. We moved all over the UK the only foreign post was in Jordan in the Middle East. Dad was in the signals regiment so he was posted to the RAF base in Amman and we spent two years in Jordan but we had to be evacuated because of the Suez crisis of 1956 we were given half a day to pack then we were all flown out on transport planes to Cyprus. Dad was a troubled man. I can't separate whether it was a result of a difficult childhood or a direct consequence of being a prisoner of war, or both. Dad was still having nightmares in the late 1960s, my mum used to tell me. He used to get up at 2 am and have a cup of tea and Mum would tell me he'd had another nightmare that night. But he had no help offered. I think it was the generation that felt they had to sort things out for themselves and there was no help anyway. He was on sleeping tablets for a while but whenever he tried to talk about 'why' to the doctor, he'd just give him more tablets. Dad was an avid reader so we'd go to the library every week and he would take out four or five books about the Second World War, principally the Far Eastern war or India, and I'd go with him and became an avid reader too. He liked being on his own. But as I say I can't separate whether this was due to his fractured childhood or because of being a Japanese prisoner.

One thing I noticed was that Dad didn't have many close friends. I realised in time that was driven by the fact he saw too many close friends die in captivity. It was mainly from disease. Some people were beaten to death or beheaded but the majority were from cholera, beriberi or infections or malnutrition.

Dad explained the diet was just a bowl of polished rice and that some prisoners went blind because there was no B12 in the diet. This meant that Dad was strict about food. Under no circumstances were we allowed to leave food on a plate on the basis that he'd have given his right arm for half of the food we had in front of us. And if you didn't eat it, the plate came back the following day with the same food on.

He just could not settle. It was only after his death that we found out why he'd been moved so much in the army. It hadn't been because they'd been working him too hard. We discovered he'd applied for every single post, wherever it took him. It was then we realised how restless he was. He couldn't stop. He wanted to be forever busy, as if he was running from something. We were reluctant to ask a lot about his time in the camps but every so often something would come on the news or in a newspaper and he'd talk about it. He said that one thing he noticed when he was held at Changi Jail in Singapore was that some people just gave up and died, he did not. The Allied prisoners were held at Changi before being moved up to the Death Railway. He said he took it one day at a time, and he gave me that advice in life: do your best, take it one day at a time.

Dad said that one day towards the end of the war the prisoners heard that the Japanese had planned one day in 1945 where all the POWs were going to be executed. But when the atomic bombs were dropped on Japan and they surrendered, the war ended three weeks earlier than that set date for executions. So Dad knew he'd missed his own execution by just three weeks. He talked about that time when the war ended, when the camp guards suddenly had to stop being camp guards and hope the prisoners didn't beat them to death.

When Dad came home to Britain, the country was in the throes of post-war rationing. Dad was abused in a shop once because he had extra rations. That made him very bitter after all he'd been through. He was also bitter that they got no compensation. He passed away aged 68, just before the government gave Far East prisoners of war a compensation payment. He missed it, and had spent his life feeling no one really cared about what had happened in the Far East.

My mother didn't talk about it much but did say that Dad had nightmares. She said at times it had been very difficult to live with him because sometimes he'd just go into a complete silence. Little things that made him so restless and unable to settle. Dad never had many close friends mainly because we moved around so much we didn't have time to make any.

My brother has been to the death railway and subsequent to that we've found Dad's service record for being a Japanese prisoner, how many camps and where they were; we know he got moved around and on the railway the camps moved with it and went further north.

## JAPAN AND THE FAR EAST

The railway of course was never finished. Most of it was abandoned after the war anyway as it was only designed to carry Japanese troops from Burma up to the Indian border.

When Dad died in 1985 of a pulmonary embolism. I went to his funeral. It's sad to say that the only other people there apart my mother, me and my brother were a couple of representatives of the local Far Eastern POW association. He was a member of FEPOW but as far as I'm aware, he'd go to one or two meetings then did not go again. There were three old blokes who were ex-prisoners, nobody else. He'd just never let anyone else get close.

The only other piece of advice Dad gave me was this: whatever you do, always stand by your decision, don't run away, be a man. He was tough. Tough to have survived. Dad was immensely proud that I went to university but it was a mixed thing. He wasn't very communicative and when I went to university in Cardiff he was in Shropshire. He didn't take me in the car but delivered me to the railway station in Shropshire and never once came to visit. 'You're 18, stand on your own two feet. Get on with it,' he said. As I loaded my trunk on the train he said: 'I'm glad you're going.' He wasn't the best communicator. I think he was trying to say he was proud of me setting out on a new life. Now when I read about all the diseases the POWs suffered in the Far East – beriberi, cholera, jungle sores, losing teeth – I don't know how Dad coped. He didn't have many teeth left when he was liberated but he had coped with so much else. Now I think about Dad a lot. I have a wonderful picture of him astride a horse in the 1930s because they were trained to ride before the war and he told some interesting tales of the horses. I'm very proud of my dad and admire the strength of will not to give up under the harshest of conditions. He was a strong character but all his pain was internalised. What grieved him most was that the Far Eastern prisoners of war were not properly recognised during his lifetime.

Many prisoners of war had not had an honourable time in captivity. A need to survive in harsh conditions had led some inmates to turn on

# THE TRAUMA OF CAPTIVITY

their own. One case was heard of Major Cecil Boon who was charged at a London court martial of aiding the Japanese while held prisoner. Boon had been a dancing champion before the Second World War and when taken prisoner, had become the Chief Administrator Officer by the Japanese. His responsibilities involved the overall administration of the prisoner of war camp Sham Shui Po. Major Boon had a network of spies in the camp who would inform him of anything going on, which would then be passed on to the Japanese. In his defence at his court martial after the war, Boon said that the prisoners of war would be better being punished by him than the Japanese. After twenty-two days of court martial, Major Boon was acquitted of all eleven charges.[9]

Another man who was a prisoner working on the Death Railway was Thomas Goodwin. His son, Kevin Goodwin, said he was a gentle, quiet man who was only occasionally able to talk about his time in the Far East but that he did spend some time at Roehampton Hospital after contracting tropical diseases.

## 'Dad said: Whatever you do, don't use creosote. It's what we had to paint the sleepers with and we were naked and it burned our bodies like hell'

Kevin Goodwin, son of Thomas Goodwin, prisoner of war on the Death Railway

My dad's name was Thomas Goodwin. He was with the Bedfordshire and Hertfordshire Regiment. He was called up and originally he spent his time in Britain during the invasion scare when people worried Germany might invade us. Eventually, he was shipped out to South Africa and then from there to India. I've got some photos of him in India. And then from there, disastrously, he was shipped to Singapore.

Dad was born in 1919, so he would have been around 23 when he was captured when Singapore fell. He was single and hadn't met my mum at that point. When he was in the prison camp he got friendly with a Sergeant Kimber, and when they came home he said to my dad: 'Come and meet the family.' Sergeant Kimber's sister ended up becoming my mother!

My mother had two brothers, Uncle George and Uncle John. George actually died in the camps in the Far East so my mum married my dad and looked after him, but had the loss of her brother in the Far East as well.

First my dad was taken to Changi prison then to another camp called Kanchanaburi. After that, I know he was in Thailand and he worked on the railway. That's all a bit sketchy as it's just from conversations I had with him. He was a prisoner until the end of the war.

I was born in 1957 so that was ten years after they were married. I'm not sure why there was that delay in having me. I don't know if that was any bearing on what happened but by the time I was old enough in the early 60s to realise Dad had gone through something special, he'd very much come to terms with it.

I talked to other family members, including my dad's mum who lived with us, and she said the first ten years had been very difficult for Dad. When he got shipped back to this country, before meeting my mum, he spent time at Roehampton Hospital being treated for various disorders he picked up in the jungle. He'd had malaria quite badly and hookworm which he eventually got a very small pension for. And I think he was helped out by the authorities. He also had occupational therapy. He made a beautiful blanket and we had that for years he'd made during his time in hospital. My mum always praised the Salvation Army as they were very helpful and they certainly leant assistance to him during the early days.

When he returned, he was very thin, emaciated. Like so many, he was not shipped back immediately, they were kept out there a bit. He was built up quite quickly once back in England. I think what helped was that my dad came from a very tough background. He and his brother were both out of the east end of London, Bethnal Green, and they were tough guys brought up in abject poverty so although the cruelty was something terrible in the camps, they were used to hunger and their ability to adapt to things was very helpful in pulling through.

But when my dad got married, Mum told me it was difficult first of all. Dad would have quiet spells. He was a very placid guy but he'd have his quiet spells and I remember being a kid and being told: 'Leave Dad alone. He wants to be quiet a while.' I think things built up in his mind and he needed time to settle down a bit.

By the time I was born I think the worst of his illnesses were over but the psychological trauma was always with him. I think he was able to subdue it a bit but he would talk about it if you asked him. It's strange, but he would suddenly raise things out of the blue. I remember when we bought our first house, I said I needed to sort out a fence and get some creosote for it. He said whatever you do, don't buy creosote. 'Back on the railway I had to paint the sleepers with creosote,' he said. 'And we'd stand there naked and get creosote on your body that would burn like hell.' Another time, I said: 'Do you want Marmite on your toast?' And he'd say: 'No! That's what they used to give the ones who didn't have long left to live in the camp. You can keep your marmite.'

When we were on holiday I was a teenager and we went to Poole or Bournemouth and Dad wanted to do fishing. He bought some cheap fishing outfits and this group of people were walking along. They were Japanese students. They went up to Dad quite innocently and Mum recognised it and could see Dad – she could just tell something was wrong. Thankfully Mum acted fast and she wandered over to the students, pulled them to one side, explained the situation. They said they were ever so sorry and carried on. Afterwards Dad said: 'I'd have thrown the bastards in the water!'

Dad was never violent but he did suffer terrible nightmares. When I was still at home I'd hear him moving around downstairs and he'd been sitting downstairs drinking a cup of tea, a cup of 'gunfire strong sweet tea with a drop of brandy in it', he called it. He said: 'That bloody Jap's been after me again.' He had terrible dreams of being chased by a Japanese soldier. I think they were with him the rest of his life. Mum told me sometimes she'd wake up and her legs would be covered in bruises where he'd been 'running' in the night.

Dad got a pension for hookworm and was regarded as a small disability pension because it was an ongoing thing rather than an injury. It lives with you all your life. The actual hookworm is removed from your body but you get after-effects of itching and weals on your back. He would ask me to scratch his back and he had marks and wheels as an after effect.

My dad died quite young. I was in my 30s when he died in 1991, aged 71. His health had started to deteriorate quite rapidly in his mid-60s and eventually he just died from heart failure. He'd been a heavy smoker and there was no way he could give up. He arranged to meet one of his old comrades and this chap came down from east Anglia and poor dad had a heart attack the day the man was visiting. Whether the trauma of memories brought it on, talking about things, and that really upset him, I don't know. He died a couple of years later.

I have his wallet that went through the war with him containing a program of a play they put on. But I think when they first were captured things weren't so bad so they had the time and energy to put a play on and do some entertainment. Dad played the part of a mason in a performance they did. I also used to have some Japanese occupation money he'd brought back from Malaya. That's really all I've got of him.

There was also an old newspaper cutting from the *Hackney Gazette* which highlighted his return from the war. There's a photo of him in India leaning on a cannon and pictures of him and my uncle before my dad went out to the Far East. I've got a picture of Dad in the mid-20s and he looks like a Dickensian child in rags, he was so poor. But he was given a scholarship to go to Grammar school but it was only partly funded and my grandparents couldn't afford to pay for books

# THE TRAUMA OF CAPTIVITY

so he'd left school at 14 and worked for Cable and Wireless as a messenger boy, carrying messages within the buildings of Cable and Wireless. Then he was called up and when he came back and was well enough to go back Cable and Wireless kept his job open. He went back for a week or two but couldn't stand being in an office so my grandad, who worked for the council, let him work with him so he trained as a plasterer. So going from a clerical, academic job he went onto plastering, and he was a very good plasterer and bricklayer but it was outside and that suited him, he couldn't bear to be cooped up.

When I was 8 or 9, Dad ran his own business building and decorating and he'd knock up half a ton of cement by hand and I had a go myself and it half killed me! He was only slightly built but strong as a lion. I'm convinced the hard upbringing helped him get through. He also had a good friend in the camp as well and I remember my mum telling me that you needed a friend. If you didn't have a good friend to look after you when you were ill and to reciprocate you would go down, and funnily enough my mum was convinced that's what did for my uncle cos he was a solitary guy and she was convinced he never had much help. But he was helped by his friend out there. It was something a lot of prisoners did. They buddied up. The surgeon who was in his camp was fantastic and saved so many lives and towards the end, they'd run out of anything and had to trade for medicines and had no anaesthetic.

This doctor was [effectively] sent back to Napoleon's time and would operate without any anaesthetic and limbs being removed. How on earth this doctor got through it, I do not know. He saved so many people.

Later on, my dad would get worked up saying it's disgusting because he was given a BEM – a British Empire Medal, which was a step down from an MBE – and Dad would say angrily: 'That's what they give lollypop ladies now.'

There was very little information assimilated to the ordinary soldiers in the camp. Dad knew there was a radio somewhere hidden by an officer but they were very careful not to spread anything in the way of new information because that would give a clue to the Japanese. So they only got very old information; I remember dad saying they had some idea the war was coming to an end one day when they got up as normal and the Japs had gone and there was no one there, the camp was deserted. And I think they were like that for several days and a group of American soldiers liberated the camp.

Dad said that the Japanese had a thing about Parker pens – they liked British made stuff. And what they used to do was try and trick the guards into trading food or whatever, they'd get an old pen and scratch parker on it to convince them it was a parker pen.

We used to go to the Far Eastern POW reunion dances and they were very jolly occasions. They were good fun but eventually they faded away as people get older. In 1957 the film *Bridge on the River Kwai* was made. We'd moved to Norfolk from London and Dad took me to the cinema in Cromer to watch it. I'm not sure what he made of it, but it didn't bother him. I can't watch it now.

Initially I remember Mum telling me that Dad would never have anything Japanese in the house. That was the rule. But as time moved on and we started getting more and more Japanese imports it was hard to avoid it. I think he come to terms with it. My first motorcycle was a Yamaha! He was happy with that though. I did try to convince him to buy a Datsun but he drew the line at that.

Despite everything, he was a kind man. He never raised his voice. He never laid a finger on me. It would just be a stare, and a muttering of 'Come on, boy', and that would be enough. I only remember him losing his temper once and I was absolutely shocked because I'd never seen him so angry. He was working for the council as caretaker in some flats; I was into car repairs and had a garage round the corner and dad was watching me put this car back together again. He was watching me put it together and this council official turned up and all of a sudden he absolutely exploded, using words I'd never heard pass my dad's lips before. I don't know what set him off, that's the only time I ever saw him lose his temper.

Dad's gone now. I wish I'd asked him more.

But of all these stories, nothing was written down, and you lose it. It's all lost. It's so sad.

I hate to use the word lucky but when I read about how other poor devils never came to terms with being prisoners of war, I realise how lucky we were that Dad coped the way he did. He really was quite a well-adjusted man. Just Dad.

## 'My father worked in a mine and never saw daylight'

David Reader's father Stanley Reader was a merchant seaman on a ship that was sunk during the Second World War and was taken prisoner

My father, Stanley, was born in 1913 in Barrow in Furness, a port town, and a lot of the unskilled men went into the merchant navy. My grandfather and two uncles had also been in the merchant navy so there was a lot of peer pressure on my father to join.

He married my mother in 1941, but before my older brother Malcolm was born in 1942 Dad had set sail for Calcutta, where he joined the fateful Empire March. He didn't even know he had a son until he had been a POW for one year and received a Red Cross letter, and didn't meet Malcolm until he returned to England from Japan in 1945.

My father's ship was in the deep South Atlantic during the war, 170 miles off Tristan da Cuhna, a group of islands between South Africa and South America. Dad had been in Calcutta and the destination was Brazil to pick cargo up. Sadly that ship was sunk by the German raider *Michelle*. Dad told me that he remembered crew trying to get to the ship's gun and being machine gunned by the Germans. He fell into the water and was grabbed by something which he thought was a shark but it was actually an African stoker who pulled him up into a lifeboat and saved his life.

## JAPAN AND THE FAR EAST

He remembered more gunfire before they were captured by the Germans. Instead of them taking their prisoners to Germany however, they sailed around the Cape of Good Hope to Singapore. There my father was taken prisoner and taken to Changi prison.

As a young boy, I remembered Dad not speaking a lot about Changi. But gradually he did let some things slip.

Dad had had a tough life in a tough town. He was one of eight children so he was already toughened up to a degree. I believe his character already steeled him and he had an attitude of 'it's tough, but you've got to get on with it'.

From Changi, my father was transferred on a 'hell ship' to Hakodate on the North island of Japan and then sent to Kamiso, a cement factory that still operates today.

My father was very lucky because the Japanese Colonel in charge of POWs was a humanist, who spoke good English and so Dad told me there was not as much violence for the sake of it. But Dad did tell me he had nose problems for the rest of his life because a guard hit him in the face with his rifle butt, simply because he hadn't bowed respectfully. There was a sense of casual brutality. Although Dad acknowledged it was not as bad as the treatment of those on the Burma railway.

Over the years Dad would tell me things he remembered, like the local women – who had nothing but would risk their lives to slip bits of food in to the prisoners. He was given a bowl of rice a day and in one letter home he wrote of how they'd slaughtered a pig for Christmas – but it had to be shared between 150 prisoners.

A number of men in the north island died but mainly through disease. After this camp, my dad was sent to another camp at Bibai where he had to work in a coal mine where he worked in complete darkness and never saw daylight.

He was there four months before in September 1945, the guard came in and announced: 'Gentlemen, I'm pleased to tell you the war is over.' My father told me there was total silence and then a huge roar of happiness. They returned home slowly so that they could be rehabilitated.

My early memories of him are as any normal ordinary dad. He had beriberi and malaria which plagued him for life. He also had to have a number of operations on his nose where he'd been hit by the rifle. I remember as a child in the 1950s I'd see Dad shivering in his bed from the effects of malaria and our doctor would have to come around and give him quinine

When I became a teenager, Dad told me more and showed how he could count in Japanese. He could also say phrases in Japanese that he'd heard a lot, such as: 'Don't let the campfire go out, or you'll get hit!' He even taught me to count to ten in Japanese.

My father was a strong man physically and on his return he was able to build himself up to work as a docker and seaman again. But his temperament afterwards was calm and for every problem he'd say: 'there are worse storms at sea'.

One of his friends survived all the years in the camp and then got hit by a cricket bat back home and died. Dad reflected on how random it all was, that you could die of something seemingly so mundane after surviving life in a POW camp.

Although Dad would answer my questions, it was never a very big conversation which I think shows part of the mentality of that era as well. I'd overhear him talking to mates or my wife's father, who had been a soldier in Italy. I think he got some relief from talking to other men.

What he would tell me about was the brutality, the toughness, the sickness, the emptying of the latrines. He made jokes about things like when you're carrying the buckets of slop on a bamboo pole: 'Make sure you're not at the back!' I believe it was that humour that got him through.

One thing I noted throughout his life was that my dad didn't have that deep hate which I know some of the prisoners understandably had. He had no animosity towards his captors.

He carried on being a seaman and docker but got an industrial disease in his lungs and died in 2000 aged 86. Dad was mentally acute right to the end and I believe he was lucky to get out of Changi and be sent to the north island of Japan and not the railway, avoiding that death cult they had there. I think he experienced a more benign environment. He was lucky.

David Reader is rightly proud of his father and his ability to cope with all he had endured. Perhaps Stanley Reader's strength equipped him to cope with civilian and family life on his return. But while some fathers were able to have relationships with their children, some simply could not adapt to caring for a child. One case is that of Margaret Kiernan whose father was captured when Singapore fell and became a prisoner of war in the Far East from 1942 to 1945. Margaret had been born in 1940 and her father was called up just a few weeks later, meaning he left as a new father who had barely got to know or bond with his baby. This, she explains, made it all the harder for him to bond with her at all when he returned.

## 'My childhood was decimated. One day Dad walked past me in the street and didn't even acknowledge me.'

Margaret Kiernan, daughter of Harry, prisoner of war in the Far East for three years

I was born in Manchester in August 1940 to young parents who enjoyed life, wearing nice clothes, going to the cinema, the theatre and music, collecting records and my father even had a drum kit which he loved playing.

Soon after I was born my father was called up to the Army and after a spell of training at Woolwich Barracks was shipped out to Singapore, he had only just arrived when it fell to the Japanese. He was first imprisoned in Changi jail and then moved on to work on the infamous Burma Railway. One can only imagine what a

# THE TRAUMA OF CAPTIVITY

shock that was for him, he was of slight build and not one of nature's soldiers. For some time my mother did not know if he was dead or alive until odd postcards arrived saying he was alive, 'being treated well and working for pay'! Of course that was not the case as we all well now know.

The next time I saw my father was in 1945. I was rising 5 and starting school, so much time had passed and having spent the war with my mother and grandmother suddenly there was this strange man in my life. Obviously he was very damaged from his experiences, he was very withdrawn and really did not connect with me. He had bad nightmares and would be shouting in the night which frightened me a lot, he also had a couple of recurrent bouts of Malaria. He could not bare any waste at all, especially food, because as I now know he had existed on a handful of rice a day plus anything they could lay their hands on, which resulted in me as a small child being made to sit until my plate was cleared, which was impossible for me as I had a small appetite, which resulted in me having nightmares about 'food on my plate', and I became scared of him and anxious. My mother finally had to speak to our family doctor about it, who managed to speak to Dad about it and explain that I was a small child with just a small stomach and could not always eat everything, which did eventually persuade him to leave the situation alone. At this time, where I had once been a happy child I became a tense and anxious one with a distant father who never hugged me or showed me any direct affection.

On reflection he had left a newborn and returned to a child and had missed out on watching and being involved in the normal development process and he seemed unable to make that transition, it seemed that I was the one that had to make the adjustment.

At that time so many children of my generation had fathers who did not return from the war so we were told that we were lucky to have one and so we accepted. The following years were quite difficult, my father was unable to settle in a job, he would often start a job but would walk out. Relatives on his side of the family who were staunch

## JAPAN AND THE FAR EAST

middle class and hard working found this impossible to comprehend as PTSD was not really known then and they gradually drifted away from him. He never talked about his experiences to anybody, army friends came to see him a few times to persuade him to attend reunions but he always refused, I think he just wanted to forget it. One day Dad walked past me in the street and didn't even acknowledge me.'

Just a couple of times he talked about things, he could not forgive the Japanese for their cruelty, one day out of the blue he told the story of a fellow POW who had gradually tamed a local monkey which became like his pet; when a Japanese guard found out he ordered the monkey to salute him and when the monkey didn't he beat the poor thing to death. While in the camp he converted to Catholicism because of a Catholic priest who was also there and was a great comfort to them, the priest made my father a rosary out of knotted string which I still have to this day; my mother was already Roman Catholic and on his return they always went to church together. I have to admit his hatred for the Japanese never really faded; he did say once that apart from their mistreatment of POWs, their cruelty to the local Malayan and Thai people was just as bad. We never had a single Japanese made item in our house, no Japanese TVs crossed the threshold of our front door, always Ferguson or other British make.

So I grew up with all these tensions and not really having a proper father. In later life he grew more mellow and once I had left home to carve my own path my parents enjoyed a quite steady life, taking their little holiday trips to Wales that they loved and without me being there they could return to the coupledom that suited them. My father died of Motor Neurone disease in 1986 age 74 and my mother in 1998 age 87 which meant that they failed to receive any of the compensation that was given to ex-Japanese POWs which was sad.

A few years ago I found some memorabilia of my father's war experiences; it turned out he was actively involved in a concert party at some point in time and there are handmade program's with

# THE TRAUMA OF CAPTIVITY

fantastic illustrations of the all male cast, these are very precious and as a family we are uncertain what to do with them.

As for my own life, after travelling abroad I joined British Airways and flew as Cabin Crew for a number of years before getting married and having my three daughters, I now live in Berkshire and apart from my three daughters, I now have two little granddaughters. It's strange to say on reflection I noticed that whenever my parents came to visit us here, which they did every summer, I would hear my father talking to my daughters a little bit about his POW experience, something he never did with me, it seemed to skip a generation, maybe other people have experienced this too, I don't know.

War is a terrible thing, it ruins peoples lives; not only did it ruin my father's life, it also damaged mine. I never really had a proper father and I guess there are deep psychological problems below the surface; only recently, when we were in a restaurant, my daughter said to me, 'Mum do you realise that whenever the waiter brings you your meal you always say "Oh! I'll never eat all that."' She said, 'Mum you don't have to eat it all!' Now I realise that I subconsciously go back to my childhood where I did have to finish everything on the plate., When considering voluntary work in recent years I chose SSAFA, a charity that helps service families who need support in some form or other. I did voluntary case work and fund raising for ten years, the choice probably influenced my own experiences.

To finalise: what happened, happened! It's been said that it was a culture difference, that the Japanese considered being taken prisoner was a dishonourable thing and that's why they treated them so badly, but the Japanese have never to this day apologised for their many atrocities and the many lives that were lost and ruined.

Margaret's father was not alone in his feeling that men returning from the European prison camps were given more time and shown more interest than the men returning from the Far East. This resounding feeling echoes again and again in the stories of the children of Far East prisoners. But because of this, and the lack of understanding of the cruelty they had experienced, these men often had to internalise how they were feeling because they had no one to talk to.

As a woman feeling that her father could not connect with her, Margaret Kierney is not alone. Another daughter is Chris Ramsbottom, whose father Kenneth was a prisoner of war in the jungles of the Far East. Before he left as a 19-year-old soldier, Kenneth was known as Sunny Jim because of his light, happy demeanour. When he returned, Chris explained he was a different man and was mentally abusive and controlling towards her and her mother.

**'He had flashback and got me and Mum pinned up in the corner of the kitchen with a carving knife cos he thought we were Japs.'**

Chris Ramsbottom, daughter of Kenneth Barratt, prisoner of war in the jungles of the Far East

My Dad was Kenneth James Barratt and he was born in 1922. Everyone called him Jim – Sunny Jim because of his sunny personality. But then the war started. Dad's family greengrocer shop took a direct hit from a bomb which inspired him to sign up.

He joined the Army just after his 19th birthday. He was sectioned into the RAF and was one of the first to be trained in radar. He was sent over to do operations in Burma.

He told me stories in segments which meant I had to piece them together, but he explained that he was shot down and his plane landed on Christmas Day 1943 in the jungle. He was only 21.

After he crash-landed he escaped his plane and was sitting on a tree stump eating a dried biscuit and feeling sorry for himself. He said he was thinking about how it was Christmas back home and his family would be eating goose when he heard a noise in the jungle. He grabbed his rifle and shouted: 'Halt! Who goes there?'

## THE TRAUMA OF CAPTIVITY

And then a little woman in a green uniform pushing a tea trolley arrived who said she was with the WVS – the Women's Voluntary Service – and she gave him a slice of Christmas cake and a proper cup of tea. He thought he was hallucinating, seeing a woman with a trolley in the jungle, but it turned out that the WVS had set up their first outstation in Rangoon and he'd landed on it.

During my childhood Dad didn't talk much about what happened so it was hard for me to piece together what took place. He told me he spent a long time in the jungle and he didn't get back to the UK until 1948 because he was ordered afterwards by the British government to stay in India and help with the partition there. He only made his way home in 1948 working on merchant ships, gradually getting nearer and nearer home.

I was an only child and I remember Dad had malaria which kept recurring. Mum would try and explain as best she could to me. He didn't sleep well and I'd often wake to hear him shouting and yelling. When I was 9, he'd done it again and I asked Mum the next day: 'Was Dad all right last night?' She explained that he had nightmares most nights and that was how it was.

He was depressed all through my childhood and would go into sulks for days. I'd have to be the go-between between him and my mother. I'd be forced to wait outside my father's room and then take a message back to my mum. I soon learnt he didn't really want a girl, he'd wanted a boy. So I tried to be a tomboy growing up. He'd give me presents of trains and cars, which I enjoyed. But he treated me like the boy he wanted, not the girl I was. He became distant.

Once when I was 8, Dad had a sudden flashback and completely changed. He grabbed a carving knife and had me and Mum pinned up in the corner because he thought we were Japanese.

From age 12 I barely spoke to him except for to say goodnight. There was no physical abuse, but there was mental abuse. I realised as I got older that Mum suffered the most from his mood swings. He was very controlling. She worked all the time because he couldn't due to bronchitis. Mum was a very traditional woman, very nurturing and yet she still went to work. Dad stayed home but he hated her having friends and only gave her £4 a week for housekeeping – for forty years!

It affected my life greatly. At 15 I took an overdose because I was so unhappy at home. I felt I'd screwed up. I let friends down because Dad would never let me out of the house.

Mum showed me a photo of Dad just after he'd joined the RAF and was on basic training and he looked hopeful and happy. She showed me a photograph of him five years later and you can see the difference. He came back a completely changed personality. My father got no help with his mental health. He had some tablets for malaria, but that was it.

In time my mother basically became his carer, as well as working and giving him all the money she earned from her jobs. I had a miserable childhood and left home as soon as I could to go to university. There, I went completely wild and felt I was finally free, let off the leash. I wanted to go everywhere and meet everybody. After being in such an unhappy environment with such controlling father, it was wonderful to finally be free.

After my degree, I then worked in a college supporting women who were survivors of domestic abuse. My mum confided in me at the time – she'd had cancer and chemotherapy and had to eat with a spoon – that Dad was being horrible, mocking her for eating with a spoon. He'd say: 'Fancy that, eating with a spoon. You're an adult.'

I told her she should have left him years ago. But I gave her exercises in assertiveness that I taught women who were survivors of domestic violence. She called me a few weeks later and said it had worked – he wasn't mocking her anymore. I now see that my father was very controlling and manipulative. He died aged 82.

Dad never met up with any POW veterans. We wanted to get him help from the British Legion but he always refused. He would never talk to them. He would never buy a poppy. I think it stemmed from

# THE TRAUMA OF CAPTIVITY

him taking so long to get home after the war ended, and being forced to stay on in India. I think he was still angry about how some of the soldiers had been treated.

On one occasion in the 1990s, Dad and my mother went on a holiday to Weston Super Mare where they met other veterans. After that meeting, Dad looked and acted better for the first time. I think he must have finally talked about what he'd gone through with someone else who had been through the same.

There was only one horrific story he shared with me as I got older and that was about 'his Canadian' as he called him. He was a friend who was also prisoner of war from Canada and he and my father became close during their captivity. He told me once that this man was bayonetted by the Japanese and Dad was forced to watch.

Mum would make me watch the drama *Tenko* on TV to try understand what he'd gone through. I tried, I really did. But I never got on with him. Now that he's gone, I see how damaged he was. I still have absolutely no documents and no information as to where he was held in captivity, only that he spent at least two years in the jungle.

I never ever knew what was going through Dad's mind and now I will never know.

His experiences had a huge effect on our family life, though, and it completely destroyed my childhood.

Some POWs returned and were able to get the help they needed to carry on and reintegrate back into the family. Sadly that didn't happen in our case.

# Chapter Six

# Coming home from Japan: Compensation and carrying on

'We heard the roar of an approaching bomber and again everyone rushed out. There she was coming in low over the trees, heading straight for us. Everybody held their breath but this time there was no hostile reception. As she swooped down we could see every detail of her markings. From one of the blisters in her side, a friendly arm waved to us.

And then we really let ourselves go. For three and a half years we had waited for this. Everybody, as if moved by a united impulse, waved, shouted and laughed. A lump came into many throats. There were even tears on a few faces caused by an overwhelming sense of relief and thankfulness that could find no other expression.'

*Worthing Gazette* – Wednesday 14 November 1945

Because of the four-month delay between VE day – on 8 May 1945 – and VJ day – on 2 September 1945, many soldiers who had been prisoners in the Far East felt there was less of a fanfare for their return than those who had been in German prison camps.

VE day saw a nation rejoice with street parties. Winston Churchill declared the day a national holiday and huge crowds arrived in London to hear Churchill speak in Whitehall and to see King George VI and the royal family appear on the balcony at Buckingham Palace.

## THE TRAUMA OF CAPTIVITY

For soldiers who had been prisoners in Germany, VE day was their national party too. As banners were hung from windows and balconies and whole streets celebrated, soldiers returning from stalags in Germany might have rightfully felt a sense of elation that was tangible.

But it was not the same for those returning four months later from Japan. Yes, street parties were held, and yes, two days of bank holidays were announced. But not many people yet knew what all these men had endured. Far from the theatrical shows in German prisoner of war camps, these men had endured the barbaric treatment from a nation who did not recognise the Geneva Convention.

Years later it would be discovered that some prisoners of war were not only tortured and killed but were eaten by their captors. Winston Churchill was apparently made aware of the practise of cannibalism by the Japanese on their enemies but would not release the information. Instead such victims 'died in captivity' or were 'missing'.

Ex-prisoners returning from camps in the Far East would have seen more horrors than those held captive in Germany. Survival rates speak for themselves: the death rate in the Far East camps was 20 per cent – seven times that of the prisoners in German camps; 30,000 prisoners of war died in the Japanese camps. Alongside the brutality, cholera was the main killer, along with beriberi disease, hookworm and other gastroenterological problems – or sheer starvation.

But first the men had to get home. Repatriating tens of thousands of men was an enormous operation. The Joint War Organisation held conferences to arrange this.

> Post-armistice repatriation.
> Sir Richard Howard-Vyse said that provision had been made for the supply of comforts at the ports and disembarkation in this country for prisoners repatriated after the Armistice and that this was on a comparatively small scale.[1]

## COMING HOME FROM JAPAN

It had been thought that the repatriation of prisoners of war would be the responsibility of the Army Welfare Authorities, but now Sir Richard Howard-Vyse was raising the issue that it was advisable for others to help out in transporting prisoners home from transit camps in Europe and back to Britain. Lady Limerick, who had joined the Red Cross during the First World War and had quickly risen through its ranks to run the London Office, was part of the JWO and it was recorded that:

> Lady Limerick strongly urged that the War Organisation should take an active interest in these men who naturally looked to the Red Cross before anyone else for assistance, and she referred to Major Creighton's report on the transit camps in Italy for men released from prison and awaiting repatriation, in which he emphasised the need for these men to be given some relief from the rigid routine of camp life in order to accustom them to their impending freedom. Major Creighton had invited the men in batches to his own private house but such a course would naturally be impossible when repatriation took place on a large scale. Lady Limerick suggested, however, that we should, if possible, have welfare workers in the transit camps and perhaps staff clubs or hostels for the men. The proposal that the War Organisation should be identified with the welfare of ex-prisoners before repatriation was approved in principle.[2]

Lady Limerick, who was famously quoted for saying 'practical idealism' was the most important part of the work she did for the Red Cross, was occupied with ensuring returning men had the emotional support they needed as well as having lodgings. And she reported in meetings at the JWO that:

> It had been agreed that the War Organisation would assist, where necessary, with arrangements for hospitality for

repatriated prisoners of war who had no homes to go to during their 28 days' leave. Lady Limerick said that, for the most part, private hospitality could be arranged through the Joint County Committee for these men but certain individual cases might arise for whom no hospitality could be found.[3]

Lady Limerick – ever the practical idealist – proposed that rest houses which had previously been used by the Civil Defence Workers' Health Department should be retained for POWs who had nowhere else to go. The minutes from meetings covered seemingly trivial practical considerations that would be of huge importance and comfort to returning prisoners: that they should be given cigarettes and stamped telegraph forms ready for sending messages home; that they should be given Red Cross vouchers to get food and other supplies they needed in camps as they made their way home. A sum of £200,000 was set aside to provide services for returning prisoners of war including gift bags and money to be set aside for invalids and those who needed special diets to readjust to normal life. The gift bags to be provided to 160,000 returning prisoners of war were to include:

> 1 razor and 5 blades, shaving soap, toilet soap, toothbrush and toothpaste, shaving brush, ½ lb chocolate, a comb, 50 cigarettes, a face cloth, two books, matches, and a message of congratulation from the Chairman.[4]

If needed, 10 per cent of these men would also be provided with:

> 1 pullover, 1 suit pyjamas, 1 pair of slippers, 1 pair of socks, 2 handkerchiefs, one pipe and 2oz tobacco.[5]

It cannot be underestimated what this gift bag might have meant to returning prisoners. Not only did it provide the practical necessities they might have been denied in captivity – shaving equipment and soap and so on – but the comforts they must have been so wistful of for so long: chocolate, books, a face cloth. Those present at the JWO meetings worked hard to include, as well as practical considerations, those touches that would ensure that prisoners of war felt human once again.

In subsequent meetings it was decided that:

> Prisoners may stay in staging camps for as long as four weeks before being moved to transit camps. Prisoners in enemy camps in the British and American zones will stay there until it is time for them to go to the transit camps. The British numbers involved are at present 43,000, exclusive of about 14,000 in SE Germany.[6]

Transit camps, it was decided, would be formed near embarkation ports and the plan was that prisoners would not need to be there for more than forty-eight hours. Prisoners who were in hospital, however, would be flown straight back to Britain. Those who were not flown directly home would remain in the enemy hospitals or transferred to British and American hospitals in liberated Europe. Crucially, it was also touched upon how next of kin and family members might need to behave around the returning prisoner of war: 'The Prisoner of War Directorate at the War Office has composed a letter giving hints to next-of-kin concerning the proper treatment of repatriated prisoners of war.'[7]

What made the return of the prisoners of war from the Far East even harder was that it took so long to repatriate them. As they did return home, newspapers of the time charted their journeys:

> **Reunited On 'Mercy Ship'**
> The 10,000 ton New Zealand ship *Manowai*, first 'mercy ship' from Singapore to dock at Colombo, carried

# THE TRAUMA OF CAPTIVITY

1,000 liberated prisoners of war and 200 internees. Wife of a British gunner, Mrs Durston, of High Road, Wembley, Middlesex, told how, with her newly born baby, she was interned in malaria-ridden camp at Bahau. She and her baby survived, but she lost her father, mother and brother. Her husband, a prisoner of war in the notorious Changi prison at Singapore, was also brutally treated by Japanese guards. The couple are now reunited aboard the *Manowai* on their way home to Britain. Another 1,500 liberated prisoners of war arrived at Colombo yesterday on the P&O liner Corfu, from Rangoon.[8]

Moving accounts such as this one that appeared in the *Worthing Gazette* in 1945, speak of the incredible moment prisoners saw the RAF planes swoop over their camps, liberating them:

**Voyage Home from the Far East**
Returned POW's interesting account

**D.B. Hearle of 53 Northcourt Road recounted his story:**
A Prisoner of War in Jap hands who has just returned from the Far East furnishes a first-hand account of his many exciting experiences, a description of the voyage home from the Far East and his joy at being safe in England again. He is D.D. Heark who writes as follows: 'Like many another returned prisoner,' he commences, 'I find myself living in a new town and was interested to read my first copy of the *Worthing Gazette* list week. After a total absence from England of over eight years it is very pleasant to be back in the old country again and I am particularly glad to find that the majority of our provincial papers have survived the war, even if

they are somewhat reduced in size. In pre-war days they formed very pleasant reminders to us the Far East of the delights of English life and I have no doubt will continue to do so in the happier days that we all trust lie ahead.

It was on August 6 when we returned to camp from our daily drudgery,' he continues, 'that we got the first inkling of the good news to come, in the story of the devastation wrought by the atomic bomb. Thanks to the courage of the few brave men operating our secret wireless set, we had always managed to keep pretty well up to date with world affairs but as the months following VE Day passed without any visible signs of a quick ending to our war we were beginning to get resigned to spending another Christmas in captivity.

Then suddenly came Hiroshima, and Russia's entry into the war and Nagasaki and for a week suspense and excitement were high. As the days drew near to the 15th the tension grew almost unbearable. Many ex-POWs will tell you that this time was in some ways the most nerve-wracking of our whole imprisonment. The Japs themselves gave us no sign that the end was near. In fact, that last week they worked us harder and more brutally even than usual. And we of course dared not reveal that we knew what was going on. When the Emperor's announcement did come it was almost an anti-climax. For on the next day, and the day after, and the day after that we were paraded as usual in the morning, given our usual wretched bowl of rice and kicked and driven to work in exactly the same way as we had been for the past three years.

Naturally, everyone began wondering what had happened. The local General had always boasted that

## THE TRAUMA OF CAPTIVITY

he would never surrender and it looked as though, despite the Emperor's order to the contrary, he would carry out his threat. None of us had any delusions as to what would happen in such an event. In our weak condition and situated as we were in the middle of a defence area we had little doubt most of us, in the event of a landing, would have been conveniently liquidated. An incident that happened a few days later almost confirmed our worst fears. Ever since the Armistice the sound of a plane had brought everybody rushing from their huts, if the guards weren't near, to watch for the longed-for red, white and blue rings of the RAF. So far, though, we had been disappointed. Jap machines still patrolled the skies. Then one lunchtime we heard the unmistakable powerful throb of a large bomber flying low. Everyone rushed out. There she was, big, beautiful, wing-tips glinting in the sunshine, cruising steadily along only a few hundred feet up. Everybody flung up their arms to wave wildly but hardly had they raised them when a vicious burst of Ack-Ack fire broke out almost directly behind us ... But it proved to be our last disappointment.

Two days later, in a guarded, stilted statement, the Camp Commandant informed us that a negotiated peace had been concluded with the Allies. We knew differently but we were too thankful to enlighten them then. Anyway we soon found out the truth. From that minute on, life became just one long Christmas Day.

Red Cross parcels that the Japs had kept hoarded for two years and more, butter, milk, extra rice and clothes, were all showered on us in a last desperate effort to get us looking less like battered skeletons before the Allied troops should land.

# COMING HOME FROM JAPAN

> Almost overnight the brutal, arrogant beast disappeared. The peacetime Jap, all bows and apologies, and sucking teeth had taken his place. But nobody was deceived. Even a Japanese leopard couldn't change his spots in that short time.
>
> Shortly after this we got our first big thrill. Again we heard the roar of an approaching bomber and again everyone rushed out. There she was coming in low over the trees, heading straight for us. Everybody held their breath but this time there was no hostile reception. As she swooped down we could see every detail of her markings. From one of the blisters in her side, a friendly arm waved to us.
>
> And then we really let ourselves go. For three and a half years we had waited for this. Everybody, as if moved by a united impulse, waved, shouted and laughed. A lump came into many throats. There were even tears on a few faces caused by an overwhelming sense of relief and thankfulness that could find no other expression.[9]

Yet, many prisoners from Japan did not come home until 1946 – a year after the war in Europe was over. They returned to a nation who longed to forget the war and move on. Tables in the street heaving with party food had disappeared and been replaced by closed doors and hard rationing. Previously celebrating families were now hungry and poor, abiding by their ration book to survive and trying to find work in a post war economy.

Any prisoner returning from a foreign camp during war would have found life hard. But it can safely be said life would be much harder for those returning from prison camps in the Far East, and not just because their treatment had been so much harsher.

Prisoners from Japan returned to a country that wanted to move on. The war was something people no longer wished to speak about.

# THE TRAUMA OF CAPTIVITY

The initial elation had worn off and now came the arduous task of rebuilding – not just homes and offices but whole lives, communities and working practices. Men who had been held captive in Germany had had a year to find their place in society again. Women had returned to the home – on the whole – and men had begun rebuilding their lives. For the prisoners returning from Japan that was all yet to come. But they were already at a physical disadvantage. Exhausting hard labour, one bowl of rice a day and their captivity in tropical jungles brought with it a whole host of illnesses, parasites and diseases that many doctors had not faced before. Some ex-prisoners gave interviews in the press.

> I produced a newspaper in Changi Prison, Singapore, during my internment there. I still have, and treasure, the complete file of 220 issues, record of a most unpleasant experience. Every issue had to be 'chopped' by the Japs before publication and the last one, in October 1943, never came back: it had been submitted coincidentally with a raid on the prison by the Military Police, alias Gestapo, in quest of wireless sets (they found three, following torture to force disclosure) and other material that did not win their approval. They took away over forty unfortunate internees to their foul cages in town. Fifteen of them died, some from violence, some from torture others from starvation and filthy diseases caused by the squalor in which they were kept, and in the prison all entertainments and such frivolities as newspapers were sternly forbidden from then on. Painful memories indeed. And let me confess that I have shed no tears over the many Japs who have been executed or given long sentences for their ferocious treatment of POWs, internees and Asiatic population of Singapore.[10]

# COMING HOME FROM JAPAN

Not only were these men haunted by what they had endured or had seen, but they had no jobs or lodgings in many cases. Huge swathes of Britain had been bombed and the country was rebuilding but housing would be a problem for years to come. One such case was that of Bill Parsons who had been a Lieutenant Colonel in Japan:

**PC 99 Wants a home**
PC 99 Bill Parsons who, as a Lt-Col in the Army was head of SEAC's Special Investigation Branch and arranged the execution of one of the Japanese General's is back on the beat again in Sunderland. Not, however, as a constable. He is looking for lodgings in the town so as to be able to go back to his pre-war job with Sunderland police force. As a lieutenant-colonel in India, he was not only head of the SIB but raised a similar branch within the 14th Army. While at Singapore, he arranged the execution of the Japanese General Shimpei on the beach outside Changi Prison where Australian POW airmen were beheaded at the General's order.

'Since I was demobbed in November I have been hunting for a house for my wife and two children who during the war were living at Pelton. I had no idea the housing problem was getting so bad,' he said. 'I told the Chief Constable I was hoping to restart as PC 99 at Christmas but I can't until I find somewhere in the town to live. I've been offered for £2,300 a house that before the war was built for £700.[11]

It was a major problem. At the end of the Second World War, Britain faced the worst housing shortage in history. A baby boom was already occurring with families who had waited for 'after the war' now having their families. That, plus the fact that an estimated

500,000 homes had been destroyed by bombing campaigns during the war, meant that the government estimated there would need to be another 750,000 new homes built. Whole streets had been destroyed and many houses still did not even have an indoor toilet.

Slums began appearing over Britain, particularly in badly bombed areas such as Coventry and London. The new Labour government led by Clement Atlee had been voted in in 1945 and proposed to solve the housing crisis by building 1.2 million new homes. Many of these would be council houses but, in order to solve the problem faster, over 150,000 prefabricated houses would be built. These 'prefabs', as they became popularly known, would house many a returning prisoner of war and his family.

> A two-bedroomed house with a well-planned kitchen that would delight any modern-minded housewife; a hot water system from the fireplace, and also an immersion heater; other up-to-date features including a refrigerator, cooker and wash boiler, all for gas, and complete to the wireless aerial – all for rent, inclusive of rates for 13s, 8d per week…
>
> Mr and Mrs Ball, and their young children Diane and Robin, seemed quite proud of their house and the interest it aroused. They moved in the same afternoon.
>
> Mr Ball served in an infantry regiment during the war, reaching the rank of sergeant. He and his family had been living in rooms in St Paul's Road.[12]

Although most council officials stressed that prefabs were only temporary, many families with returning prisoner of war men were only too glad to have a house at all. Despite so many being built, there were still long waiting lists and many returning servicemen were living in slum conditions or rented rooms. But it was a vicious cycle for many returning men: they had no home to go to but often didn't have the means to find work to be able to rent anything better. Many men who had returned from the Far East camps were badly damaged psychologically – although they and their doctors at the time might not have recognised this – and would struggle to adapt to ordinary life at home, let alone in the workforce.

> Repatriated prisoners of war, particularly those from the Far East, find themselves faced with many difficulties when the time comes for them to return to civil life – the ordinary difficulties of the civilian in this post-war world, which to them are new and strange although so painfully familiar to us; domestic problems which may have arisen during their long absence away from home, and above all the vitally important question of settling down again in their own jobs or, as happens in many cases, finding new ones more suited to their capabilities. As a result of the conditions he has endured during a long captivity, many a returned prisoner finds himself quite unable to cope with all these problems and the outcome, if he is left without guidance and help, may be disastrous for himself, his family and in the long run the country. So far as the Army is concerned, a determined effort to meet this situation has been made by the setting up in various parts of the country, of twenty Civilian Resettlement Units.[13]

These resettlement units were set up to provide a half-way house for returning prisoners of war to find work or be trained to find new work in skills they had not yet learnt. They also provided medical and dental help for prisoners too. But most importantly, they were one of the few places these men could talk about their mental health – even if they did not use those words as we do:

# THE TRAUMA OF CAPTIVITY

Resettlement scheme spreads remarkable successes:

The returned prisoner of war who thought he would find it quite easy to take up his old civilian job, and who hasn't found it quite so easy after all – may, in fact, have 'cracked up' at it – and who, besides that, finds it difficult to mix with his comrades in civil life – this is the type of man for whom the Civil Resettlement Unit is proving a godsend. There are other types too – the repatriate who joined the regular Army as a lad fifteen years ago and doesn't feel quite confident about competing with the men who have had years of training, the ex-POW whose mental state has been complicated by finding an unhappy home life waiting for him, the man who just wants to look around and find his bearings before going into Civvy Street. They have all come to the CRUs and benefited from them.[14]

The twenty civilian resettlement units around the country became so effective that the scheme was made available to any returning prisoner of war even if he had become a civilian up to twelve months earlier. Over time, the resettlement units evolved to include camp halls – where ex-prisoners could meet and talk – a stage, cinematographic projectors, and even families' hostels adjoined to the camps where ex-soldiers' wives and families could stay while the men were there.

Back in 1944, psychiatrist Philip Harker Newman had written a paper in the British Medical Journal called 'The Prisoner of War Mentality: Its Effect After Repatriation'. In it, he discussed Dr Vischer's 1919 study in which he coined the term 'barbed wire disease' and wrote that it was, in fact, a misnomer. Interestingly, Newman decided to focus not on what the man had gone through in captivity – although it was, of course, important – but how that man would adapt into normal civilian life *after* captivity.

> During this period of enforced imprisonment they have adopted a certain mental attitude – a frame of mind compatible with camp life. Dr Vischer has traced most carefully the origin of this mental attitude and discussed in detail its symptoms during camp life; he has not, however, described the symptoms after release from the camp.[15]

This was groundbreaking at a time where men were supposed to come home and 'get on with life'. Newman delved into what happened to a soldier during incarceration, and how he dealt with this impacted how he could return to civilian life:

> The effects of internment are twofold, and can crudely be divided into physical and mental. The physical effects are easily described and easily accounted for. Their treatment after release is probably a matter of good food, elementary medicine and pleasant conditions… Unfortunately this is not the case in mental convalescence where, as doctors, we tend to flounder in directing treatment. Formerly, what we call common sense was the guiding principle, and it will remain so unless some very clear and rational indication for additional methods arises. The use of individual psychological treatment for any returned prisoner of war seems to be debatable; it may carry with it a public acknowledgement of mental abnormality, which must at all costs be avoided.[16]

This sentiment of avoiding the admittance of any kind of 'mental abnormality' is a sign of the times in which post-war soldiers lived. Nothing would be so degrading as to be labelled 'mentally ill', and so psychiatrists, although finally acknowledging that imprisonment had huge effects on soldiers' mental health, had to tread a fine line of treating prisoners and aiding them, but without drawing attention to their psychological problems to the wider community. This is why Civilian Resettlement Units were so important: they were a place only prisoners or war and soldiers could go and be with people just like them. They were a place where talk of mental illness, or of nightmares, or anxiety or depression, could be raised without fear or ridicule or ostracization.

In 1945, a study was undertaken of 100 prisoners of war who had been admitted to a military neurosis hospital. According to the study, at first glance all the soldiers displayed the same traits of irritability and inability to withstand any kind of restriction whatsoever, along with restlessness, depression and in some cases paranoia. The men showed 'limitation of all interest, difficulty in making any social contacts, poor concentration, preoccupation with their own problems, and a well-marked tendency to show resentment towards anyone and anything.'[17]

Interestingly, the study found that 24 per cent of returning prisoners had developed some of their symptoms before being captured – these were called pre-capture conditions. The study found that these men already had 'marked neurotic traits' and that 50 per cent of them had a neurotic family history, 25 per cent had suffered previous nervous breakdowns and 60 per cent had shown 'pronounced neurotic traits' in childhood. Moving on to capture and life while imprisoned, the study found that 44 per cent first showed neurotic traits on capture itself, that early home life and a poor father relationship and a tendency to rebel, led to greater neurotic traits. In 30 per cent of men who had stressed that restriction was felt greater than others, 22 per cent had shown delinquency in childhood such as 'stealing and wandering'.[18]

The study found food – or lack of – was an all-consuming obsession for pretty much all the prisoners of war but was more pronounced in certain men. The study found that men from backgrounds which had included insecurity could not stand the food deprivations in a prison camp and became absorbed and preoccupied with their physical health as a result. Another group who suffered greatly as a result of food deprivation was a group of men who had placed greater importance on physical prowess – when they found they were weaker due to lack of food, they became preoccupied with never being 'real men' again.

Of great interest in the study was a mention of one prisoner of war whose fiancée wrote to him saying she had found herself a 'real man' to replace him and that a 'real man' would not get himself captured. The study claimed that similar instances like this also occurred, where soldiers held prisoner suffered guilt for being captured and received letters from women complaining that to be captured was not to be a real man. The general consensus among men who felt guilt at being captured was that a good soldier should not be taken prisoner, as well as guilt at surviving and being relatively safer than their counterparts still in the front line or involved in active battle.

When the men were released, the study found that 32 per cent of them suffered from 'release syndrome', which often included a fear of open spaces, a sense of helplessness and a childlike sense of fear of organising his own life again without the order and structure of prison camp life. Some, the study claimed, even longed for 'the monotonous security of camp life again'.[19]

In another study by Dr Newman's, published in the British Medical Journal in 1944, a prisoner's lack of sexual intercourse and lack of interaction with females was also discussed. Newman found that many men were concerned that lack of the act of intercourse itself might lead to impotence, but that the wider and larger concern was that the men would be forgotten by their women.[20]

Newman wrote movingly of how, when returned prisoners of war gathered to hear a talk from an Air Force prisoner, they reacted with most emotion to one line the ex-prisoner said: 'And chaps – the girls still love you.' He also wrote of the stages of being a prisoner of war, ranging from the breaking-in period (the most unpleasant stage, he said); the second stage, the period of convalescence, where the prisoner accepts his situation; the third stage the period of boredom; and then stage four, the repatriation period. Newman wrote that many – if not all – prisoners returning during stage four would experience 'irritability, disrespect for discipline and authority, irresponsibility and even dishonesty'.[21]

He elaborated that other extreme reactions during the repatriation period might include a fear of enclosed spaces, fear of crowds, embarrassment and quick and violent tempers. Newman was positive, however, that 'the syndrome, when it exists, should pass after six months to one year, and thus those affected should give rise to no concern.'

The 'types' of men he did give concern to, however, were men with exaggerated symptoms, or those with persistent symptoms:

> The first type is associated with symptoms of severe restlessness, irritability, emotional outbursts, acute discontent, and possibly excessive alcoholism. The second type shows chronic apathy, loss of initiative, and loss of morale and of personal drive, resulting in the inevitable appearance of more serious neurotic symptoms.[22]

Newman wasn't simply discussing the ways in which prisoners of war might be affected mentally. He proposed suggestions of how returning prisoners of war should be contacted, treated and monitored.

He proposed that every returning prisoner of war should receive a pamphlet containing advice and who to contact if he felt he needed extra help. He also suggested that an advice organisation would need to be created by medical practitioners, adding: 'Medical practitioners who have actually been prisoners of war would be of great value in these circumstances.' He suggested that a prisoner of war club should be created in all large towns in Britain 'with a population of over 100,000', where prisoners could find like-minded people who had endured the same experiences. 'These advice centres,' he wrote, 'may also be used by relatives seeking advice in handling returned prisoners.'

As these men talked, were counselled and spoke of what they had gone through, word got out of the cruelty they had endured in the Far East. The newspapers sensed the outrage against the Japanese captors as families learnt how their loved one had suffered and reported on the war criminals, as they were now known, being brought to justice.

### 'Death Railway Man Hanged'
### 'Singapore, Friday:

'Death Railway' Man Hanged Singapore, Friday: Eishan Hayashi, Korean Guard known as 'The Maggot' to Allied prisoners of war working on the Burma–Siam 'death railway', was hanged this morning at Changi Gaol, here. An Australian War Crimes Court sentenced Hayashi to death for having kicked in the stomach sick Australian prisoner of war who did not stand to attention quickly enough when Hayashi entered a hut at Niki Siam. The Australian died soon afterwards.[23]

### 'Jap War Criminals Hanged'

Singapore, Thursday: Three Japanese war criminals, including two major-generals, were hanged at Changi Gaol this morning for atrocities against prisoners of war. Major General Otsuka Misao and Major General Hidaka Mihoo were found guilty of causing the deaths of thirteen British prisoners of war, four Dutch prisoners and twenty-two civilians at Outram Road Jail here. The third criminal hanged was Sergeant Kimura Tako, who was sentenced to death for beating and torturing Australian prisoners of war working on the Burma-Siam railway.[24]

But even months after many soldiers had been repatriated, the hell of not knowing continued for those whose loved ones did not come home. So many men had died during the building of the Burma Railway, or simply of disease, that many families had to wait months before knowing the truth about their relative. One moving story was that of Mrs M. Sharpe, who was told her son had died as a POW in Singapore but then received a Christmas card in her son's handwriting three years later posted from America. She believed that perhaps the authorities had got her son's death wrong and that he was really alive.

> **'HOPES OF MOTHER DASHED: Soldier son died in Singapore'**
> Believing that he might have lost his memory, she wrote to the Mayor of Elizabeth (New Jersey), enclosing a photograph of her son and yesterday police there were combing the town for Sharpe. Her hopes were bolstered by a report from her son-in-law that Richard Arthur Brown, taken prisoner with Leonard Sharpe, had seen him alive more than three years after his reported death. Last night, however, Arthur Harry Bates, ex-soldier of the Leicestershire Regiment and fellow prisoner of Sharpe called on Mrs Sharpe. He said that as camp bugler he had sounded 'Last Post' and 'Reveille' over the grave in Changi Cemetery, Singapore, of her son who died in Roberts Hospital in March 1942 of malaria and dysentery.[25]

Ironically, Changi Prison was the place many war criminals in Japan were held while they awaited trial. But meanwhile in Britain, a specialist tropical diseases clinic was opened at Roehampton for returning POWs from the Far East. Many treatments were trialled there including a ten-day treatment plan to help bring relief to the patients returning from Japanese internment camps who suffered malnutrition, emaciation, beriberi disease and more; by 1950 there were 150 beds.

John Baxter was treated there for hookworm – a parasite that feeds on the blood in the intestines. Untreated, hookworm led to severe infections, blood loss, anaemia, protein deficiency, shortness of breath and even death.

In an audio archive clip on the website Captive Memories, he said:

> I was married in 1948 and in 1950 or thereabouts there was an alarm call all over Great Britain where they were getting an influx of POWs that were suddenly dying. They all proved to be chaps that were on the Burma railway and what it was, they got this hookworm still in their body…in the Far East particularly in rivers in Burma there's this tiny parasite that gets into any orifices in your body and it hooks to the membranes inside your stomach and feeds on your stomach. Anything you eat is diminished, all the vitamin content of what you eat is destroyed by these things and they're progressively eating your stomach lining away…
>
> What they did was they instituted a two-week intensive check-up and treatment for anyone that had been in the Far East and they were calling them in batches of fifty … they did the same thing as they'd done in the Queen Alexandra hospital seven experts in every branch and you went through the mill. It was a really thorough check-up and it was so exhausting – we were there two weeks – and every other day we had to rest. The local Women's Institute had to take us chaps that were well enough to walk about … to local activities. At the end I still hadn't had any treatment, not even an aspirin.

## THE TRAUMA OF CAPTIVITY

Then we had to go through another trial at Roehampton and there were another seven experts there and you were lying on this table and you're stood there and they said how do you feel? I said, well, I'm a bit exhausted. Some of it involved physical tests to see what you could do, others were drugs and things and whatever the tests were, you were given things to drink and you had to give routine samples of urine. It was a twelve-hour session of being treated by various surveys related to all these different complaints, whether you'd had them or not. I didn't have beriberi but I still got the check, which was sometimes some horrible stuff you had to drink and the next day they took your blood tests. You were always being punctured and tubes stuck up here and everything that so you were a bit washed out by the end. But it was offset by the very good service you were getting there, the comfort, the facilities inside the hospital and the fact that [the WI] were running coaches everywhere to the West End to see shows and visit places of interest in between. When I faced this tribunal at the end, they said, 'We've got a list of all your complaints here and we've given you all the specific remedies and so forth in this test that we give.'

And then they said, 'We can't find anything wrong with you.'[26]

Fergus Anckorn was another soldier taken prisoner in Singapore. He survived a massacre in a hospital by playing dead. He was interviewed and in an archive audio of his story by Captive Memories, he said:

I was in the battle of Singapore and I was a gun driver and I had to get a new gun, our gun had been hit. On the way back with it the Japanese spotted me from the

## COMING HOME FROM JAPAN

air and bombed me. I was blown up and the lorry was on fire, I went to open the door, my right hand hanging off. I kicked the door open and jumped out and at that moment I was shot. That was the last day of my fighting in Singapore and I ended up in the Alexandra Hospital.

While I was in there the Japanese came into the ward; they'd taken over the hospital grounds and they killed everybody. The walking wounded they took out and killed on the front lawn, then they came and killed everyone in their beds, including staff. When they came to me I had just passed out again, as I'd been doing all the time, and my right hand was on my chest and was bleeding profusely onto the floor and they thought I'd been bayonetted so they walked past me and killed everybody else. In my ward there were seventy-one of us and when I woke up there were four left alive, of which I was one. Then they went upstairs and killed some more, about 200 in total, and I woke up next lying on the floor of a Chinese girls' high school – one of fifteen survivors of the 200 odd that were killed and that was how I started my prisoner of war days. During my prisoner of war days, I was buried alive twice by Allied bombing.

One day the Japanese decided to take five of us out, for no reason at all; they just picked five of us, put us in a lorry which was most unusual because we always had to walk barefooted. They took us to the jungle, they lined us up against some trees and they got out a machine gun and aimed it at us and we waited; we stood there waiting for the bullets to hit us for ten minutes. I was very frightened. You would have heard my knees knocking from here I tell you. Then suddenly they thought better of it, they put the gun away, put us back on the lorry and took us back to camp and there we found that the war had been over for three days. And that was the end of my prisoner of war days.

I wasn't looking too good at the time and I was sent to Burma to be fattened up. Three months I was in Burma and then I weighed six stone so I was allowed to come home. About a year after coming home my health was still pretty bad in all sorts of directions particularly mentally and I found myself referred to Queen Mary's Roehampton where I ended up in the ward specifically for ex-prisoners of war far east. There I had a funny feeling all the time that something wasn't as it should be. To start with I found that we had to wear blue uniforms with red ties which were the army sick outfits which were all laundered each week and we didn't know whose we were wearing. I thought this was terrible as it was years after the war, we were all civilians and we had to dress up like this. We had to clean the ward out and polish the floors. We had a sister there I think her name was Buxter or Buxton and she was a real terror I think everyone was terrified of her including me and the consultants but she ran the ward extremely well.[27]

Fergus recounted his story on the Friends of Queen Mary Hospital website and talked of how before the war he had worked as a magician and how this kept him alive. During his incarceration in the Far East he found that his Japanese captors loved magic tricks. He would deliberately do tricks involving food the Japanese had, such as a tin of fish or a banana. After the trick, because the Japanese found the prisoners verminous, they would not eat anything they had touched and so Fergus would get the food he had used for the magic trick, quite simply keeping him alive.

Another soldier, William, who was in the 9th Northumberland Fusiliers Z Company was captured in Singapore when it fell in

## COMING HOME FROM JAPAN

February 1942. He was held in Changi prison and various others before being repatriated on the SS *Corfu* to Southampton. In an audio archive interview he said:

> One of the most difficult jobs I had when I came home was to meet the mother of two friends who lived just 100 yards away. They were both still in Thailand and both died and I had to go and see their mother and she knew they were dead or missing prisoners of war. My brother and I both came home and I had to go and see their mother.[28]

But of course, as word got around how much the Far East prisoners of war had suffered and the previous sanitised reports were proven to be untrue, the general public did finally rally around to recognise them. One such example is that of the Blackpool Prisoners of War Association who offered a free honeymoon in the city to any returning POW from the Far East.

> **'Free honeymoon for ex-captives'**
> Any Far East prisoner of war getting married on his return home can have a free honeymoon in Blackpool. All will be eligible – it is not just for local boys – and in anticipation of hundreds accepting the invitation, leading private hotels and boarding houses are being approached. Some have already agreed to give the couples hospitality in their best bridal room for a week. Blackpool branch of the Far East Prisoners of War Association is preparing in a big way for the return of 400 local boys. Their health, their future, their homes will be cared for. Wives, sweethearts and mothers are being taught how to look after those who may be suffering as a result of their imprisonment. University lecturers are to teach them to care for men suffering from tropical diseases.[29]

# THE TRAUMA OF CAPTIVITY

It was a wonderful intention, of course. A honeymoon in Blackpool at the time was not to be sniffed at. And teaching women to understand their husband-to-be's possible malnourishment, stomach and indigestion problems, inability to eat a large meal, signs of beriberi and worse, were all useful skills to learn for any family member of a returning prisoner of war. But talk of the psychological impact of what they had gone through was alarmingly non-existent. A free honeymoon for a returning prisoner of war might give a man and his bride a week of bliss. But what about afterwards? What about the nightmares? The fear of going back to work? The fear of sudden movement or loud noises or enclosed spaces? What would be the treatment for that?

Some people were asking those questions, but in an era where the words 'mental health' were not as well-known as today, it took second place to physical recovery. Of course, doctors did monitor and follow up patients they had seen, especially with regards to tropical diseases and stomach problems picked up in the Far East:

> **'British Red Cross and ex-servicemen'**
> Four years ago, many Nottinghamshire men were languishing in Japanese prison camps, their bodies wasted from starvation and ridden with tropical diseases. Last year the Nottinghamshire Joint County Committee of the Order of St John and British Red Cross Society asked itself two questions: How are they faring today? And: How can we help them?[30]

A report into the ongoing care of returned prisoners of war and how they were faring was presented at the annual meeting of the After Care Department:

> All the men and their families are grateful for the interest. Assistance has been given in some cases over difficulties

which have arisen regarding their health, employment, pension, etc. Queries have been received regarding everything from licenses to build a house to how to get food to feed an ex-serviceman's pig. Working quietly yet effectively, the department is helping more ex-servicemen who might otherwise have been 'forgotten men'. Equipment for occupational therapy, invalid foods, clothing, food parcels and other goods have been supplied to more than a third of the disabled veterans whose cases were investigated.[31]

In Nottinghamshire, the After Care Department report found that 265 fresh cases had been brought and 335 had been revisited – some several times. Social workers visited men who were in a sanitorium. But, as written in the *Nottingham Journal*, many of the men who had returned from the Far East prison camps saw themselves as the forgotten ones. Their war had lingered on longer than in Europe. Their returns had been staggered and postponed, months later than their comrades from the German camps. This notion of Far East prisoners of war being forgotten would linger on for many years and, for some, would never ever disappear.

# Chapter Seven

# Glorification versus Reality

'Colonel Von Luger, it is the sworn duty of all officers to try to escape. If they cannot escape, then it is their sworn duty to cause the enemy to use an inordinate number of troops to guard them, and their sworn duty to harass the enemy to the best of their ability.'

Group Captain Ramsey, *The Great Escape*

'I put my union jack at the front, I put my head down and played the punch drunk soldier. I could have stared in the camera and put the bird up. But the difference between reality and movies is that, in reality, they really will kill you. This idea that you eyeball your captors is rubbish. They do not allow any of that to happen.'

John Peters, prisoner of war during the Gulf War

As the world left the decade that was known for war and entered the 1950s, rationing was still in place in Britain. But although life for the average person was still very much a struggle, one area of industry was booming: post-war books and films. Enough years had now passed where artists and writers felt able to create works about the war and prisoners of war became a great subject matter.

One of the most famous films of that time – and arguably, ever made – is the film the *Bridge on the River Kwai*. Released in 1957, the film was critically acclaimed and won seven Oscars.

## GLORIFICATION VERSUS REALITY

The film was based on the novel of the same name by Pierre Boulle which was published in French in 1952 and in English two years later. The characters and events in the novel are fictional but the story is set against the backdrop of the construction of the 'death railway' and so was quickly bought for film rights, with Sir Alec Guinness, William Holden and Jack Hawkins signed up for major roles.

One major scene in the film features Colonel Nicholson (Alec Guinness) in a stand-off with Colonel Saito, the Japanese camp commander. Nicholson holds up the Geneva convention to Saito, telling him that his officers must not be forced to do manual labour. Saito grabs the book and tosses it aside after striking Nicholson across the face, much to the shock of his men.

The film follows the men as they are forced to work on the construction of the Burma Railway and how Nicholson decides that rather than refusing, by building the bridge it will give his men something constructive to do (as well as showing the British engineering superiority over the Japanese.)

The film won critical acclaim and is still to this day a classic prisoner of war film. But, like most films of that genre – and prisoner of war films would become just that: a genre in their own right – it is jingoistic, imperialist and glosses over the many horrors that we now know happened in the camps in the Far East. In the 1950s, just a few years after men returned from these camps, not much was known among the general public of just how horrific their time there had been. The healthy-looking actors, the positive attitude to building a bridge they can be proud of, the morale which rarely ever dips, are all tropes of the 1950s war film which helped boost post-war morale.

But the truth was of course very different. Many ex-prisoners of war would later complain that the film showed them as complying with their captors to build the bridge when, in fact, they were often forced to work at bayonet point, in the nude or wearing only a cloth for modesty, or at gunpoint.

## THE TRAUMA OF CAPTIVITY

Letters later revealed showed that the War Office was also unhappy with the script of the film, worrying that it would not authentically portray officers' conduct in the Far East during the war. They also believed the film would not go down well with the public. Lieutenant General Arthur Ernest Percival, who was then chairman of FEPOW – Far Eastern Prisoners of War – wrote to the War Office:

> The subsequent picture of the bridge being built under the British Colonel's directions in a most efficient manner is a very false one. It would have been very wrong for prisoners of war to have willingly done this because it would have been contrary to their duty ... Whatever may be said, either in the book or in the film by way of explanation, it is certain that a high proportion of those who read the book or see the film will form and retain an impression that this conduct was typical of that of British prisoners of war in the Far East.[1]

Lieutenant General Percival ask that the film be censored, but when that didn't happen he requested that a disclaimer be put on the film so that 'no aspersions are cast on the conduct of British troops'.

The idea that a high-ranking colonel would have encouraged his men to work willingly and with pride for the death railway must have cut like a knife to those who had endured the horrors of working there. The real life colonel in the camp that the character of Nicholson was based upon was Philip Toosey, who had been in the Territorial Army. The idea that the Japanese needed the captured troops to build the Burma railway is also fictional – the Japanese had been planning to build the railway for many years but now had 60,000 captive troops to use as slave labour.

In the film, Colonel Nicholson is kept in a sweltering hot metal hut for three weeks. When he is brought out of the hut, almost dead, Nicholson goes to Colonel Saito and agrees to build the Japanese's

## GLORIFICATION VERSUS REALITY

bridge. (Something the Japanese also objected to about the film – they did not like the idea that they were portrayed as unable to build their own bridge without British prisoners' help!)

Colonel Toosey – the real colonel – had negotiated not only better food for his men but also a day of rest. Toosey went to see the film and didn't give any major objections, but the men who were beneath him were furious as they believed the film depiction was a slur on his character. The real Colonel Saito and Colonel Toosey later corresponded and Saito said of Toosey: 'He showed me what a human being could be. He changed the philosophy of my life.'

*The Bridge on the River Kwai* ends with the bridge being blown up by commandos – a symbol debated by film analysts for many years. Was it a symbol of the futility of war after all the blood lost building it? Was it a symbol showing that the Allies had won in the end? Was it representative of destroying Japanese pride? Or was it also simply a wonderful piece of movie magic? Either way, it is not the truth. The real Kwai bridge is still standing and still has trains running across it to this day, a monument to the many brave men who died or almost died building it.

Another equally famous prisoner of war film is *The Great Escape*. This was released later than *Bridge on the River Kwai*, in 1963 and tells the story of group of Allied prisoners of war determined to escape from Stalag Luft III. Featuring the biggest names in the industry at the time – Steve McQueen, Richard Attenborough, Charles Bronson and James Garner – the film was unsurprisingly a huge success.

The story is set in 1942 and based on the non-fiction work by Paul Brickhill. The story follows the men as they plan an audacious plot for 250 prisoners to tunnel out and escape. They name their tunnels Tom, Dick and Harry, and seventy-six prisoners do escape. The plan fails, though, as fifty of the escapees are killed, either by the Gestapo on orders from Hitler himself, or they are found during their plan to escape through the Third Reich. By the end of the film only three prisoners successfully escape.

## THE TRAUMA OF CAPTIVITY

Again, this film focuses on the amazing strength of human character, of resilience and the desire to be free and working together to reach that freedom. The very theme tune, whistled by so many in all the years since, conjures up that plucky determination of the Allies to trick their German captors and be free. But in reality the escape was anything but great. Fifty of the escapees were recaptured and shot at Hitler's orders. It was a tremendous waste of life.

More importantly, while German stalag camps were not comfortable places, a prisoner had to weigh up the risks of escape versus the comparative safety of being in the camp in the first place. On the whole, British POWs were not as badly treated by the Germans as by the Japanese. Yes, they were on starvation rations in many cases and yes, incarceration by anyone in any time would be far from pleasant, but was it worth risking your life to escape when, come the war's end, and assuming your captors continued to adhere to the Geneva Convention, you had a better chance of survival if you stayed put?

It is hard to debate these things when you hear the rousing tune of the Great Escape or watch the young and handsome Steve McQueen hurdling barbed wire on his motorbike as he flees to freedom. But again this film glamourises imprisonment. It focuses on camaraderie, brotherhood, resilience – all wonderfully important traits and admirable at that – but does not delve much further into the horrors of being a prisoner of war; the worries of how they'd return to normality once they did escape, and the futility of loss of life for only three men to find freedom at the end anyway.

The true 'great escape' was one of the great tragedies of the war where fifty lives were taken as punishment so that only three could find freedom. This film's notion that prisoners of war should – and did – give up their own lives for their brothers in arms, is what might have contributed to making life so hard for returning real life POWs.

How could a prisoner who had endured life on the Burma Railway watch *The Great Escape* and feel good about his life? How

## GLORIFICATION VERSUS REALITY

could he explain to his wife, his children, his friends that life was not like that in a prison camp; that starvation wiped out any desire to escape, that the trauma of seeing a friend executed prevented any further longing for brotherhood? The 1950s and 60s – the great era of the prisoner of war film genre – extolled prisoners of war, but it also took them further and further from the truth of what really happened, perhaps making those much-needed conversations between ex-prisoner of war and a loved one even harder to broach. One can imagine a child watching Steve McQueen hurdling barbed wire on his motorbike and asking: 'Father, why didn't you do that and escape your camp?'

The simplification of life and escape from these camps in these glorified representations, to some degree, set back the discussions that should be had about the reality of being a prisoner of war and the wearing down of body and spirit.

Another famous prisoner of war film was of course the 1955 *The Colditz Story*, starring Sir John Mills and Eric Portman as the infamous 'bad boys' always planning another escape. The plot follows the lives of the POWs in the high security Oflag IV-C, also known as Colditz. The men are told early on that escaping is forbidden but begin planning their escape. The main protagonist, Richmond, plans an escape dressed as a German in uniform but is arrested and put in solitary confinement. Another soldier Winslow escapes but is found and returned to Colditz.

The men live with the frustration that no British officer has managed to escape, until they hatch another plan to be staged during a show held in the castle's theatre. The film ends with two men escaping and four men being recaptured. Days later, the recaptured prisoners receive a postcard that their friends, Reid and Winslow, have escaped over the border to Switzerland. The film is a high-action work with little reference to the ennui and loneliness of being a prisoner of war. Still, it is a favourite with many and up there with *The Great Escape* as one of the great prisoner of war films of all time.

## THE TRAUMA OF CAPTIVITY

There are many other great prisoner of war films to discuss but the two most famous are *The Colditz Story* and *The Great Escape* so have been included here. But one major marking in both these films is the jingoism and jaunty approach to escaping, without a lot of reflection on the difficulties – or horrors – of being a prisoner of war. For the returning prisoner it must have been a very strange experience to see these films on the big screen just a few years after being released from a camp. For some it might have brought back memories they did not want to face. For others, it might have been laughable at how inaccurate some parts of the films were.

And for others, witnessing the heroics of Steve McQueen or hero-like soldiers escaping Colditz, did it make them feel inadequate that they had not escaped or tried to? Prisoner of war films often have, by the very nature of their genre, the idea that the Allied soldiers are cunning and clever and are able to bamboozle their hapless German guards. Was this funny to a returning prisoner of war? Or offensive?

The popularity of the prisoner of war film genre waned in the 1960s as people longed to forget war and forge on with a new decade. As people learned to live under a cold war, rather than an active one, the public feared nuclear devastation far more than another outright war. As weapons changed and developed in their ferocity and a nuclear stand off between America and Russia began, war, it seemed, would change forever too. It seemed unlikely any Allies would ever live to see such combat as seen in the First World War or Second World War again.

And yet, in 1990, Britain went to war in the Gulf. After the Iraqi leader Saddam Hussein invaded Kuwait, the UN Security Council and NATO formed an alliance and began Operation Desert Shield, in a bid to protect Saudi Arabia who feared they might be next. The offensive campaign, Operation Desert Storm began in January of 1991. The Gulf War was the first war Britain had seen in its newspapers, with its own soldiers and airmen being deployed, for years, certainly not since the Falklands War of 1982. With the Allies' superior technology and air power, it seemed impossible anything could go wrong.

And yet it did.

Although the Falklands War had seen Jeff Glover, a Harrier pilot, held captive as a POW, the Gulf media coverage was by comparison more fervent. One of the most famous and notable Western prisoners of war of recent times is John Peters. A fast jet pilot employed in Operation Desert Storm in the Gulf War of 1990–1, John Peters had trained for ten years – costing £1m – and was then a flight lieutenant. On the very first day of the war, John Peters and his navigator John Nichol climbed into their Tornado jet and set off from Muharraq Airbase in Bahrain and flew across the Iraqi desert. Their job was to drop eight 1,000lb bombs on Ar Rumaylah airfield, southeast of Baghdad. But, as they reached their destination, flying at just 25ft and at 650mph, the bombs failed to release.

The men instead dumped the bombs in the middle of the desert. As they were beginning to return to base, the unthinkable happened. The Tornado plane was hit both by a surface to air missile and anti-aircraft artillery. The Tornado was damaged and both men had to eject. After the frantic noise of the explosion and emergency warning clangers, they landed in the middle of the Iraqi desert where John recalled in interviews it was 'deathly quiet'. John Nicol, the navigator, had landed 100m away from Peters. He came over to John with his parachute and famously said: 'This'll be the Iraqi desert.'

John Peters suffered minor concussion, a cut eye and badly injured his knee. But while initial thoughts might have been of relief to be alive after ejecting, the men's fate was about to get so much worse. They were in broad daylight in flat desert with no one around. They made radio calls to base explaining what had happened, that they were down and safe, and began to evade. But then they saw people on the horizon. As John Peters recalled in a television interview: 'That is the time that you can feel your heart pumping and you think: what do we do? You feel your eyes widening, you've gone from a big Tornado with lots of power, guns, missiles and bombs to two little pink bodies in the desert.'

A group of Iraqi soldiers ran towards them brandishing rifles. The two RAF men lay still with nothing to hide behind, hoping for a miracle, when suddenly a shout went up.

The group of soldiers began spraying the ground around them with bullets from AK47s. Peters said in an interview soon after: 'John [Nichol] said: "Shall we go out with a bang?" but I said: "No, there's always hope."'

The men gave themselves up. The Iraqi soldiers reached them and began hitting and punching them. The melee continued until an Iraqi officer stopped them from beating the men further. Peters and Nichol were thrown into a vehicle and driven back to the airfield they had attempted to bomb and were paraded in front of soldiers. Afterwards they were taken to Baghdad in cuffs and blindfolds, before being handed over to Iraqi interrogators.

The two Johns were separated and were both beaten by groups of men. John Peters recalled the beating ended after a time and he was returned in darkness next to John Nichol, still blindfolded, before both men were separated again. John was asked: 'Pilot or navigator' by his interrogators.

He tried to reply: 'I cannot answer that question,' but before finishing his sentence he was hit around the head with a baseball bat that catapulted him the floor. They grabbed him by the hair and threw him back to the chair, before asking again: 'Name, rank, pilot or navigator' before being hit to the ground again and again. He was beaten with baseball bats, rubber truncheons, his hair was set on fire, burnt with cigarettes, threatened with gang rape … suffering days of violence. Peters kept to the rules of capture only answering his name position and rank and was beaten whenever he didn't answer a further question. His interrogators hit his eye again and again he recalled: 'They kept on hitting my damn eye and it was already closed anyway. I just thought it's OK, as long as they keep hitting

## GLORIFICATION VERSUS REALITY

that because it was so swollen at that stage. It was just a balloon full of water...'

John recalled in interviews after his ordeal that he began questioning whether he was weak. 'I found myself talking to myself,' he recalled. 'Trying to say, no, you haven't got me yet ... trying to take myself out of it.' As his ordeal went on, John Peters realised it was not going to stop. His daughter Toni had only just been born and his son Guy was a toddler. Then one of the interrogators began stamping on John's injured knee and he let out an involuntary yelp which gave the interrogators an advantage because they finally realised his weakest point, and began kicking and stamping on his knee again and again.

It was then, after hours of torture and beatings, John finally said: 'Pilot'. After a day or two more, John was accused of being a war criminal and his captors told him he must go on national TV as a war criminal or he would be shot. John refused. But each time they slapped or hit him, adding: 'You'll never see your wife or children again.' They put a gun against his head and John knew then he would have to go on TV or be killed.

What happened next made headlines around the world. John Nichol and John Peters were paraded on television in their RAF uniforms. John Peters sat before the camera, his beaten and bloodied face visible for all to see. He looked down, his swollen eyes proof of the beatings he had endured. John was given the chance to send one message home. He said: 'Helen, Toni and Guy I love you. Mother and father...'

After the television moment, John and his navigator were thrown in isolation cells where they were kept for seven weeks. During that time, John suffered regular beatings and abuse. He was starved. Newspapers in Britain and around the world all led with the story on their front pages. The *Daily Mail* wrote: 'What has he done to them?' with pictures of Nichol and Peters on television. The *Sun*'s front page featured: 'Bastards of Baghdad – Hang Saddam Low and Slow.' For the weeks they were captive, they were rarely out of the public's minds. Despite twelve airmen in total missing, it was Nichol and Peters that were first and foremost on people's lips.

Their images, bruised and bloodied Peters and defiant Nichol, were in everyone's minds. They were the ONLY prisoners of war of the generation, it seemed.

For seven long weeks, the men were held captive. They spent most of that in total isolation, only being removed for further beatings and abuse.

It was only when an Allied bomb hit the building that everything changed. Finally, the prisoners could communicate with each other under their cell door hatches and realised they were both still alive. Four days later, John Peters was released and taken to Jordan after forty-seven days imprisonment, mostly in isolation. As his plane touched down in Cyprus and he stepped off, he was confronted with the fact that his face had been on the front of every newspaper around the world.

John recalled that before the war, 'Helen was with John and I, when we talked about the last time the RAF operated in the Gulf being the 1920s when the Bedouins threatened that if they ever caught an RAF pilot they would 'cut their balls off and sew them up in their mouths'! Obviously, the first thing I wanted to do in Cyprus was phone Helen. The first thing she said was: "Have you still got your balls?"' She was testing me to see if I remembered the previous conversation, my response would show her if the same 'person' would be coming home. One of John's biggest fears during being a prisoner of war was whether his two-year-old son Guy would forget him. But instead, on his arrival back on his base in Germany, his son ran to him shouting: 'Daddy, Daddy!' and he knew his son had remembered him.

From that moment on John Peters and John Nichol became household names. John Peters recalled being thrown from total darkness into 'bright light'. He was interviewed by national newspapers, television stations and journalists from all over the globe. His photograph appeared internationally. The men's magazine *FHM* even did a photo shoot with him in his uniform in a 'Top Gun'

## GLORIFICATION VERSUS REALITY

style pose. He had lunch with Princess Diana, a private audience with Prince Philip and shared a stage with Nelson Mandela. From unknown fast jet pilot, John Peters was now a symbol of the war, a symbol of hope and survival. He was the prisoner of war we had all cared about, and all prayed would come home.

But his story did not end there. In fact, a new life of coming to terms with his experience and adapting to this new life was just beginning. He had survived; he had endured unthinkable torture and abuse – but now he would have to decide what he did next.

John was unable to go anywhere without being recognised. If he entered a pub, he got a standing ovation. He never had to pay for a drink or for a meal. Grown men came to him and cried on his shoulder. Friends quizzed him as to what he had endured. Mothers embraced him in public – he was everyone's son, everyone's brother. His Squadron Leader, Pablo Mason, had spoken to the press during John's imprisonment and broken down at his guilt to reporters. Now he said it was 'bloody marvellous' that he was alive and well.

But for John, adjustments had to be made. He had had to adjust from life as a fighter pilot to being a prisoner of war, to living in complete isolation in a dank, cold cell, to now celebrity attention. He was flown around the world, appeared as a guest on television shows, taken for dinners, a VIP at award ceremonies. The contrast could not have been more stark. One moment a damp cell in an Iraqi military police base, the next, flying first class and meeting celebrities, heads of state and members of the royal family. If an ordinary prisoner of war found adjusting to life at home difficult, how on earth was it for John Peters?

**Anyone could go through what I went through: humans are meant to survive**

Interview with John Peters, ex-RAF fast jet pilot squadron leader who was taken prisoner of war during the Gulf conflict

# THE TRAUMA OF CAPTIVITY

I joined the military not because I was ever very militaristic but because I wanted to fly fast jets. When I was captured in 1991, I went from being an unknown pilot to mass media attention with 'that image' known around the world. A lot of people ask is it better to be an optimist or a pessimist in a traumatic experience. The answer is neither. Sometimes being the pessimist really works because it makes one assess the dark side and plan against it. But overall, optimism is hope. This aligns with the Stockdale Paradox. Admiral Stockdale was one of the highest-ranking and longest serving POWs in Vietnam. When asked about captivity, in a desperate situation, being tortured and in pain, how does one get through? His response was: it's a paradox. He explained that one must balance the brutal reality with enduring hope. If one remained in either mindset, one would give in. 'You must never confuse faith that you will prevail in the end – which you can never afford to lose – with the discipline to confront the most brutal facts of your current reality, whatever they might be." — And that is the paradox. If one totally remained solely in either one, you'd give up. And I resonate with that.

Because if you look at the beatings, the pain, the humiliation you would give up. If that is, indeed, the rest of your life. To endure as a prisoner of war, I 'looked beyond the walls'. I planned the rest of my life. But you can't go completely live in enduring hope because you're not dealing with the brutal realities, you will give in. But if you live just in the brutal realities without enduring hope, you'll give up as life is not worth living. The paradox is how you balance those two facets off: facing the brutal realities and enduring hope. And that's what I did. My way of coping with being a prisoner of war was acceptance – to accept the present, to accept what's happening to you. Acceptance requires you to acknowledge your fear and then, (my key word) to forgive yourself. Two minutes ago, is a waste of time as a prisoner of war. Therefore, dwelling on things like 'I should have, I couldn't have, why wasn't I stronger, was I weak, did I let myself down?'... all those insecurities are past-focused, and you will destroy

## GLORIFICATION VERSUS REALITY

yourself. You must accept the here and now. Be in the present. And to do that, the root to acceptance is to acknowledge your emotional response to a certain event. Why? Because we assign a meaning to something and, under pressure, in an environment that elicits a highly emotional response, that meaning is invariably wrong. So, if you're feeling really upset, that distress makes you stay in the past. You must acknowledge that emotional response. And then ... You must forgive yourself.

I'm not religious but it's forgiveness. Because until you forgive yourself, you cannot be in, and accept, the present reality. Otherwise, you remain in the past, in blame. And, as a prisoner of war, why do you need to be in the present? Because you must learn to adapt rapidly to new circumstances. This is your new world. A world that is constantly changing. If you can't adapt to the now, then you will fail. Acceptance opens you up to learning rather than blaming yourself or staying in the past. After I was captured, when my captors forced me to go on the TV, I felt I had failed. As an officer, you're not meant to give in; you are just not meant to do that. You are meant to have the character to endure. I had not given in. But I just wasn't prepared to die for just answering one question because, to be honest, that was stupidity. I expected to be shot after I had been on the TV. Before I went on, they put a gun against my head. I thought, this is it, I'm going to die and everyone is going to think I didn't fight. They gave all the prisoners a script to follow. I never stopped fighting.

My only pride was I didn't do the script. We didn't see each other on the TV because they isolated us, so for all I knew I was the only one doing it. I just felt that would be the enduring image my children would have of me: that I was a weak, traitor, failure of a man. But what you see in the recording of me on the TV, was acting. I turned my arm forward to make my Union Jack badge prominent at the front. I put my head down and played the punch-drunk soldier. I could have stared into the camera and put the bird up. I could have said, 'Fuck you!' But the difference between the reality and movies is, in the real case, they literally will 'fuck' you. The idea that you can eyeball your captors is bullshit. It is all about authority and power. They do not allow any of that to happen. What you saw on TV was acting. I wasn't a broken man. I played what you saw. What it really was, was absolute defiance.

If I was going to die, I wanted to show I was under duress and forced into it. I got away with it, mumbling and murmuring. I played as if I was punch-drunk. They put the mic higher and higher up on a pile of books. Eventually this Iraqi major pulled me out of the chair in front of the camera, literally nose to nose and stuck a gun in my eyeball and said: 'I will shoot your balls off if you don't do this.' He was compelling and not joking! I only became aware of Admiral Stockdale on my return, but formed the same conclusions, albeit less erudite! My mantra was 'Accept the brutal realities' and 'Look beyond the walls.' In other words, captivity is a mindset: if you focus solely on the walls, the beatings, the degradation, and humiliation: if your life is the wall only four feet away, then you would give up. So, look beyond the walls. Look beyond the limitations, your fears, and the present. I planned the rest of my life in captivity. I accepted the brutal facts and looked beyond the walls. And that entails compartmentalising your emotions. Of course, I thought about my wife, Helen, and my children, Guy and Toni. Guy was 2 years old; Toni was 6 weeks old when I went to war. But I could not let that sensitive, soft part of me in because it exaggerates the brutality, and I would have given up. You cannot afford to be soft in a brutal regime. You're living in a hard world.

So, my idea of enduring hope is keeping those emotions at arm's length ... as a driver to my future but not allowing them into my present. If you pull that softness into you, it will exaggerate the brutality of the reality. But you need hope to drive to endure and survive. Since my release, I view life with the same paradoxical thinking. I went from black box to white light. The black box of captivity was pitch black most of the time. I was in a violent environment in which I was

## GLORIFICATION VERSUS REALITY

trying to hold on to who I was and my sense of identity despite the circumstances. Simply, I didn't want to die disappointing myself. But when I was freed, I was suddenly exposed to white light – the world's press, all the bulbs, all the lights. Suddenly you cannot see beyond the end of your nose. I was 29 years old and suddenly catapulted into global awareness. It was highly politicised, and everyone suddenly wants a piece of you. It is overwhelming, confusing and frightening. The same mindset prevailed: deal with the reality and look beyond this to maintain a sense of self.

That is how I dealt with fame … it is not real. It is perception. I could not live up to the perceptions, so you define yourself, hold onto your own identity. Just like captivity. It is all about identity: two sides of the same coin. Upon release, first I was taken to the RAF hospital in Cyprus. There, I phoned Helen. She picked up the phone I said: 'Hi, it's me.' And her first question was: 'Have you still got your balls?' And we laughed. I made a joke back. Later, she said that the moment I made the joke back she knew I was fine. When I got home, everyone was stunningly nice. I do understand why the generation who fought the Second World War did not talk about it. Because everyone had a war experience. Everyone lost a son, or a father, or a brother. It would be cruel or impolite; all such a question would do is resurface pain for someone. But our case was very different. So, few people in our generation had experienced war. And suddenly there are these two POWs paraded on TV – John Nicholl and me. We had no idea in captivity, but we were global news. And upon our return, you couldn't shut people up! There were no such limits. No one had a filter.

There were thousands of questions every day, including from friends. Everyone was desperate to know every detail: the torture, the violence, how did you deal with it? Were you raped? Everyone wanted to know that. Concurrently, everyone was overwhelmingly emotional: people were crying and shaking when they met us, men and women hugging us. Chief executives of major companies were

## THE TRAUMA OF CAPTIVITY

breaking down when they shook my hand. It was like a tsunami of emotions. It is overwhelming and confusing, awkward, and amazing in equal measure. In my head, I was thinking: What the hell is happening? What has happened? How the hell do I live up to this response? I cannot live up to the attributes being placed on me. People were shaking when they met me, treating me like porcelain. I felt unbelievably responsible to best represent all my friends who had been to war. Do the right thing. And therein, after being a prisoner of war, you have to deal with this 'fame' experience the same. You must manage yourself and not be defined by the circumstance. It is about your sense of identity.

Of course, others want to understand; they wish to dismantle, to define. Everyone wanted the story. Behind closed doors, I was fine. In fact, from then on and until today I have not lost one wink of sleep from being a prisoner of war. If you were to ask Helen and my closest friends 'What did the Gulf War do to John?', the answer would be, it's made me more confident, maybe a little more emotional. But don't we all become more sentimental as we get older. Therein you become less aggressive and more reasonable. Also, I was exposed to literally thousands of letters and conversations from people sharing their own stories of abuse or painful experiences. One cannot retain the same 'military mindset'; my world had shifted, the perception of me had changed and one must adjust to this new order. Of course, sometimes, it can be irritating. Everyone's asking: 'Are you OK?' As if I had been damaged in some way, when in reality, you think: 'Hang on, actually, I've just dealt with a situation I'm really quite chuffed with how I dealt with it. Why does everyone assume I'm damaged?'

To my chagrin, because she is probably right, Helen explains that despite being a fighter pilot, I was too impressed by others; thinking everyone was so much better than me. I am quite liberal and would acquiesce to a strident, stronger, personality. I would flex, as I believe there is always another way. So, at times if you really pushed me, I would have backed down. But the Gulf changed that. I realised

## GLORIFICATION VERSUS REALITY

that my flexibility in the past was an advantage. I always thought the more assertive characters in the military were better, but I found that in captivity my flexibility was a strength. After the war, one of our most senior POWs said: 'You led us through the war.' I replied: 'What do you mean?' I was in a concrete box with a metal door being systematically beaten and starved to death. I could do nothing. But he said: 'It's not what you did or did not do ... Each time we got blown up, when we were talking, it was as if you were talking over a garden fence. And the way you talked, we trusted you and believed we could get through it.' I hadn't realised it at the time but that was how I was during my whole time in captivity: through the starvation, beatings, humiliation, and abuse. I reminded myself that it didn't define me. And I never wanted to die disappointing myself. The truth is, when you're 1,000 miles from anybody who likes you and your captors take you into a little room. And you are naked. And they put a gun against your head, and you can hear the mechanism click and you've got a quarter second before your brains are blown out, you gain a clarity and honesty. The simple fact is: 'I'm going to die. And no one is going to see me die.' So, it doesn't matter whether you cry like a baby, whether you shit yourself, whether you eyeball them. The simple fact is I am going to die. And in that moment, you do not want to die disappointing yourself. There is no one left to impress.

There is a truth when people say your life flashes before you. I believe that to the extent that your brain goes into hyper-think, and in a quarter of a second you think 1,000 things. Afterwards, this pulse of energy expands out. The realisation of all those thoughts become real. The real strength about captivity is you have space to explore that. And in that moment, I thought: 'I don't want to die disappointing myself. I know why they're hurting me. However, a nice chap I am, I've got a beautiful wife and stunning kids. But ... so has my captor. And now his brother has no legs because someone like me has come and blown them off and we're fighting over the price of a barrel of oil and he's defending his country.

# THE TRAUMA OF CAPTIVITY

So even in those split seconds, I accepted the reality. In uniform, I was a military pilot who dropped bombs and applied violence to political intent. And so, of course they responded violently. Doing what they were doing. But I didn't want to be defined by that. I wanted to define myself as to who I am. And the word I chose that I wanted to die like was 'nice'. I know English teachers say never use the word 'nice', it's a meaningless adjective. But I was brought up in a family where everyone said we were a nice family. Yes, you could use other adjectives such as decent, hardworking, respectful, pleasant, but these are all encapsulated in the word 'nice'. In those moments where I thought I would lose my life, I thought I don't want to be defined by the circumstances or by hatred, I want to die as me. Nice. And so the hammer goes down. Click. Nothing. But that experience provides real confidence. It becomes definitive. You know who you are. So, when everything else is taken away and you've only got yourself to rely upon, that gives you a huge sense of self. And that's where you gain your confidence.

Before we went to war, we had a lecture on combat stress to prepare us. But none of us ever dreamed we'd be captured. Then, when I got back, we were put into groups and given counselling if we needed it. After my release, after I was reunited with Helen and my children, Guy and Toni, I was offered counselling. You don't really have the choice. They offer it and you say yes. And I realised that I didn't really want or need it. I felt I had coped. And that is like the majority of people following an extreme, traumatic event. We cope. In fact, most people cope, around 75 per cent of people cope! Often, immediately after a traumatic event, the media write that people are suffering from PTSD. They may be suffering from PTS. We must separate post-traumatic stress (PTS), from post-traumatic stress disorder (PTSD.) The two are connected but different things. For those who experience PTS, you might cry, not want to eat, be emotional, and maybe this lasts maybe a week, two weeks, six months but you are coming to terms with the extremity of the experience you went

## GLORIFICATION VERSUS REALITY

through. That is post-traumatic stress – PTS. It's perfectly reasonable and about 23 per cent of people who have been through a traumatic experience suffer PTS. So human beings are built to survive! The majority learn to live with, and deal with, trauma. And yet everyone talks about PTSD.

In the military, PTSD emerges, on average, around fourteen years after the event. This is a disorder whereby the individual cannot function – post-traumatic stress disorder. Hence, fourteen years or so after an event, why it is so difficult to unravel what precisely caused it, or which precise moment you began to unravel. It might not actually be when a soldier sees his mate blown up. It might be something smaller, seemingly innocuous whereby some responsibility is assumed for that in their subconscious, the soldier then might think his friends died because of him. PTS and PTSD are very real. We should help people who experience it. But the danger is that we say everyone has PTSD when they do not. Most people cope.

Did the moments I talked in one session prevent me dwelling on something? Maybe. I cannot tell. Following the Falklands War, they found that giving someone therapy can actually send someone into therapy! Consider someone has been through something very traumatic, they have a coping mechanism and are dealing with it. Asking 'are you OK?' can elicit the response, I thought I was OK… but maybe I am not? So, therapy can send a person into therapy, even if it's not required. Not everyone needs therapy. It is fundamentally appropriate and important that we provide help to those that need it. But let's not start from the assumption that everyone needs therapy following extreme events. I was offered the card of a psychiatrist. The offer to chat was there if I wanted it, but despite what I'd been through I didn't feel I needed to.

What they did do, however, was brief everyone around me on my squadron to be prepared for how I might behave. They were briefed: 'John, might behave this way, or that way.' So, the reality was I ended up walking around in a bubble because everyone was prompted on how I might behave. Meanwhile, I was also getting used to domestic life. After being in a black box for weeks, I went to the supermarket, stood there and literally went: 'Wow!' You see things differently. You stand outside and you smell the air. You notice things, like pale sunlight. And you get that joy of life, the heightened senses. But for me that lasted about two weeks and then I was back to worrying about my phone bill or my credit card.

I was aware I should have been looking at life in a fundamentally different way after being a prisoner of war. But normality returns quickly. I was 29. You've still got to buy a house, still got the rest of your life ahead of you. The dramatic difference was that I went from 'Average Joe' to headline news: the Press, journalists, flash bulbs and TV appearances. Every mother hugged me as if I were her son. An Air Marshall crying on my shoulder, saying he was a sham, saying: 'You know what it is to go to war. I have spent thirty-five years in Service and do not know – how do I lead people now?' I had my fellow airmen and women coming up to me and asking me the most personal things about captivity. And sharing their own intimate life stories.

Everyone wanted a piece of me. I was invited to a rape crisis centre to talk to eighty women who had been raped. I got tens of thousands of letters arriving from people who had been abused. It was suddenly the most overwhelming sense of responsibility to best represent those people who did not have the level of attention I had. My life became paradoxical. One moment back to normal life flying on the squadron, the next, five-star hotels. I lost count of the times I had lunch with Princess Diana. I shared a stage with Nelson Mandela. Introduced Heads of State. I spoke in front of the Queen. I had a private audience with Prince Philip. I was given the key to a city in Los Angeles. All hugely privileged experiences. I accept that. But no more or less deserved than all those who served. I had all this attention and expectation, but the reality is that you cannot live up to the attributes that people think you have.

## GLORIFICATION VERSUS REALITY

The whole experience is wonderful, flattering; unreal and misplaced. And in between all that was a young, perhaps shallow, fast jet pilot trying to balance responsibility and vanity, trying not to believe the press. You cannot believe what the press writes about you because you cannot live up to it. I was as flawed as anyone else. You become defined by 'being the prisoner of war'. Balancing the attention with the reality: you are not that funny, not that attractive all of which is projected onto you because you've been given this 'story'. It took me two weeks to get used to it. It lasted around two years. And then it just stopped. When the attention stopped, it was a bit of a damp squib. Before, people had given me standing ovations in pubs and it was impossible to buy my own drinks. Then one day I went into a pub and no one stood up. No one bought me a beer. And then the invitations stopped coming. You don't get that invite to the function at the Guildhall in London. And suddenly you realise your story is over. But again, it is just a transition. Just as it was hard transitioning from dark cell to bright bulbs, I had to transition to normal life again.

I did an MBA, left the RAF. Started a business. And I realised I had changed but perhaps for the better, in that my experience had made me stronger. Do you know how much confidence this experience gives you? 'What's the worst you are going to do to me now? Are you going to kill me?' I was fortunate because the experience gave me a significance and a voice. It led to me starting my own business – helping people define and find great leaders for their businesses. Concurrently, I am on the speaking circuit. I am surprised that people still want to hear my story – over thirty years later. Now, thirty years on from that war and my capture, if you ask my wife and kids about me, they'll tell you I'm just a boring middle-aged man going through all the things a boring middle-aged man goes through. I'm no different to anyone else.

People ask me how I feel towards the men who held me captive. Andy McNab of Bravo Two Zero famously said if he ever met the people who captured him, he'd shoot them. My response: I'm ambivalent. My thinking is this: I was there to drop bombs on those people. So, when they caught me, what were they going to do to me? Yes, there is international law and, yes, of course POWs prisoners should not be interrogated and tortured. Let's reverse the power balance and give my captors the power. Let's give them twenty years of education, a million pounds worth of training. Let's put him in a £30m aeroplane. Then let him fly over us and drop bombs that blow your kids' legs off. Then they end up in your garden and they have information that can save your other child who's in the military. What would you do to them? One becomes philosophical.

My story has given me a wonderful life. I have been very lucky. People still ask me how I got through my experience as a prisoner of war. How come I was not damaged by the experience. It took me around fifteen years to find an answer. And it goes back to my earlier comment on dying as a 'nice' person. My mother and father raised me in a very ordinary household. I got into grammar school and all my parents instilled in me was to 'go to university and see the world'. All I can remember of my childhood is: it was nice. I say that I had a normal upbringing. But as I get older and you hear so many stories of damaged childhood, maybe I was privileged. I had a sense of being loved and a sense of being worthwhile. The result of this? As a POW, I realised I had no real self-respect or self-esteem issues, which now, to my view, comes from being loved as a child. Apart from that I think every human being is built to survive. I have no special attributes. And yet, all we hear in the media is post-traumatic stress disorder. The narrative is always on the negative. We never hear about post-traumatic GROWTH. Someone coping with a circumstance does not seem to be news. It is a better headline that someone has been permanently damaged. But that's not my story. I repeat, I've not lost a wink of sleep over what happened to me. And that is my belief for most human beings. When we go through pain, what do we tell our children afterwards? We tell them what we have learnt. And that is how I got through captivity and how I have lived my life. I didn't dwell on post-traumatic stress but on living and growth.

John Peters went on to run a very successful business and also works as a public speaker. He insists that anyone could have survived as he did and adapted as he did. He believes we all have the human capacity to survive against the odds. Yet, every prisoner of war, from every time, must face his re-entry to society in his own way, with his own psyche, with his own support network, or lack of.

So what made John Peters adapt so well to coming home? He insists that he has no special attributes, that he has nothing any other prisoner of war did not have. And yet, not many of us could have faced what he did and come out so positive and 'ambivalent' to one's captors. But what John's story does show – and what it echoes from other eras of prisoners of war – is that the desire to survive is indeed universal. However long it took to adapt on his return, however difficult or easy it might have been, each prisoner of war who survived did return to their homes, their families and jobs. Although in many cases, trauma still haunted them or they were blighted by physical ill health for many years, if not for life, that desire to survive of which John Peters speaks was universal. It spurred them on. Whether it was the 1920s, the 1940s or the 1990s, these prisoners of war had to return to a life they had left behind and that, in each case, had changed massively while he was away. For the prisoners of war in the First World War, they returned to a world where societal ideas of role and class had been shaken forever. For the huge masses of prisoners of war who returned after the Second World War from German camps, or the horrors of the Far East death railway, they too had to retake their roles as father, husband and worker. Whichever era it was, these men had to do the same thing: adapt and survive.

And although their forms of battle, their uniforms, their technology and access to mental health services differed hugely as the decades passed, they all at heart suffered the same types of experiences: unjust incarceration, brutality, starvation, humiliation and the new world they had to face on their release and return.

Now, as worldwide peace and international security is as fragile as ever, one wonders if prisoners of war on the scale discussed in this book will ever be seen again. Technology, many experts argue, will one day make foot soldiers obsolete in future battles. Drones will replace fighter pilots, artificial intelligence ultimately could replace the regular foot soldier. So will prisoners of war be something we will not see again in future artificially-enhanced robotic conflicts?

Whether we do or not, the stories of past prisoners of war must not be forgotten. Not least because we must be reminded of man's inhumanity to man when one is the prisoner and the other the captor in times of war. As my great-grandfather was asked by his German captor: 'Why did you come here to fight your cousins the Germans?' and he replied: 'Because I was made in England', shows politicised conflict soon overtakes any feelings of kith or kin. Prisoners of war have always been at the mercy of those who hold them and the Geneva Convention proved to be a weak deterrent in the Second World War, at least in the Far East theatre of war. And yet, the accounts of family members of prisoners of war show that the same experience can affect someone in very different ways. Is it due, as John Peters says, to upbringing and having the self-esteem that comes from feeling loved as a child? Or, as others argued, was it the very lack of self-esteem from a harder childhood that made their father steely enough to survive starvation, forced labour and degradation and make it home?

It is a question I would not attempt to answer.

May all those who lost their lives as prisoners of war and all those who came home rest in peace.

# Notes

## Chapter One

1. A Memory of Solferino, J. Henry Dunant, p.16
2. ibid, p.20
3. ibid, p.21
4. ibid, p.24
5. ibid, p.26
6. ibid, p.35
7. ibid, p.35
8. ibid, p.57
9. Walsall Free Press and General Advertiser, Saturday 17 December 1870
10. Annex to the Convention: Regulations Respecting The Laws and Customs of War on Land – Section I: On belligerents – Chapter II: Prisoners of war – Regulations: ART. 4, Convention IV, The Hauge, 18 October 1907
11. ibid ART. 5.
12. ibid ART. 6.
13. ibid ART. 7.
14. ibid ART. 8.
15. ibid ART. 13.
16. ibid ART. 18.
17. ibid ART. 20.
18. A Memory of Solferino

# THE TRAUMA OF CAPTIVITY

## Chapter Two

1. www.hants.gov.uk/rh/archives)
2. *Dundee Evening Telegraph* – Monday 4 October 1920
3. *Sussex Agricultural Express* – Friday 18 June 1926
4. *Dundee Evening Telegraph* – Tuesday 1 November 1927
5. *Daily Herald* – Wednesday 9 June 1920
6. *Reynolds's Newspaper* – Sunday 10 October 1926
7. *Manchester Evening News* – Tuesday 25 September 1923
8. *Birmingham Daily Gazette* – Friday 03 August 1923
9. *Burnley News* – Wednesday 25 July 1928
10. *Todmorden & District News* – Friday 23 July 1926
11. *Boston Guardian* – Saturday 27 May 1922
12. *West Middlesex Gazette* – Saturday 05 November 1921
13. *West Middlesex Gazette* – Saturday 05 November 1921
14. *Hampshire Advertiser* – Saturday 05 June 1920
15. *Hartlepool Northern Daily Mail* – Tuesday 05 May 1925
16. Convention relative to the Treatment of Prisoners of War. Geneva, 27 July 1929

## Chapter Three

1. International Red Cross – icrc.org; Le Comité International de la Croix-Rouge aux Belligérants
2. https://www.yourlocalguardian.co.uk/news/4639987.shell-shocked-wwi-soldiers-labelled-pauper-lunatics-in-croydon-asylum/
3. Steven Cherry, Mental Healthcare in Modern England: The Norfolk Asylum/St. Andrews Hospital 1810–1998 *(*Woodbridge, Suffolk: Boydell Press, 2003
4. 1890 Lunacy Act s.12; 1957 Royal Commission Report, p.87
5. Hinz, Uta (2006). Gefangen im Großen Krieg. Kriegsgefangenschaft in Deutschland 1914–1921 (in German). Essen: Klartext Verlag

## NOTES

6. Yarnall, John (2011). Barbed Wire Disease: British & German Prisoners of War, 1914–19. Stroud: Spellmount
7. https://www.thenational.scot/news/16140893.prisoner-war-letters-tell-poignant-tale/
8. https://universitystory.gla.ac.uk/ww1-biography/?id=1471)
9. The Hospital and Health Review 393 The Report of the War Office Committee on "Shell-shock."
10. ibid
11. ibid
12. ibid
13. Prisoners of War, WWI Prisoners of War in Germany & Turkey, https://www.forces-war-records.co.uk/wwi-prisoners-of-war-in-germany
14. Press Association, Friday 22 November 1918.
15. *Dundee Courier* – Saturday 14 December 1918
16. *Express* – Tuesday 24 December 1918
17. https://archive.org/details/correspondenceger00grea/page/n1/mode/2up
18. https://archive.org/details/correspondenceger00grea/page/6/mode/2up
19. Frederick O dream, Dr Wilson, Queen Square Records, 1918
20. *Lancashire Evening Post* – Friday 15 October 1920
21. *Western Times* – Thursday 15 January 1920
22. *Dundee Evening Telegraph* – Monday 02 February 1920
23. MacPherson 1923, Mitchell and Smith 1931, 320–321

## Chapter Four

1. *Montrose Standard* – Wednesday 9 May 1945
2. Ripley and Heanor News and Ilkeston Division Free Press – Friday 04 May 1945
3. *Derby Daily Telegraph* – Thursday 26 April 1945
4. ibid

5. *Leicester Evening Mail* – Saturday 21 April 1945
6. *Dundee Evening Telegraph* – Tuesday 29 December 1942
7. *Eastbourne Herald* – Saturday 7 December 1946
8. *Torquay Times*, and South Devon Advertiser – Friday 15 February 1946
9. *Derby Daily Telegraph* – Thursday 19 April 1945
10. ibid
11. ibid
12. ibid
13. British Prisoner of War Relatives' Association, no 58, February 1945 https://ibccdigitalarchive.lincoln.ac.uk/omeka/files/original/501/22597/MCurnockRM1815605-171114-025.1.pdf
14. British Prisoner of War Relatives' Association, no 58, February 1945 https://ibccdigitalarchive.lincoln.ac.uk/omeka/files/original/501/22597/MCurnockRM1815605-171114-025.1.pdf
15. BMJ, 22 April, 1944
16. BMJ January 6, 1945
17. ibid
18. *Eastbourne Gazette* – Wednesday 25 April 1945
19. Neurosis in Escaped Prisoners of War, 1946, Jeffrey/ Bradford
20. ibid
21. ibid
22. ibid
23. ibid
24. ibid
25. ibid

## Chapter Five

1. *Daily Record* 21 February 1942
2. *North Devon Journal Herald*, 9 July, 1942
3. https://www.independent.co.uk/news/world/japanese-troops-ate-flesh-of-enemies-and-civilians-1539816.html

## NOTES

4. *Dundee Courier* 8 September, 1945
5. *Dundee Courier* 8 September, 1945
6. Surgery in Japanese Prison Camps, Coates, A. E. Anz Journal of Surgery, Volume 15, 1946
7. Surgery in Japanese Prison Camps, Coates, A. E. Anz Journal of Surgery, Volume 15, 1946, p.151
8. Surgery in Japanese Prison Camps, Coates, A. E. Anz Journal of Surgery, Volume 15, 1946, p.154
9. *Yorkshire Evening Post*, 21 September, 1946

## Chapter Six

1. Joint War Office JWO- 1-1-12 p.1
2. JWO- 1-1-12 p.1
3. JWO- 1-1-12 p.3
4. JWO- 1-1-12 p.7
5. JWO- 1-1-12 p.8
6. JWO- 1-1-12 p.7
7. JWO- 1-1-12 p.9
8. *Dundee Courier* – Wednesday 19 September 1945
9. *Worthing Gazette* – Wednesday 14 November 1945
10. *Blyth News* – Monday 26 May 1947
11. *Sunderland Daily Echo and Shipping Gazette* – Friday 17 January 1947
12. *Shipley Times and Express* – Wednesday 10 April 1946
13. *Evesham Standard & West Midland Observer* – Saturday 16 March 1946
14. The Scotsman – Wednesday 13 February 1946
15. The British Medical Journal Vol. 1, No. 4330 (Jan. 1, 1944), pp. 8-10
16. The British Medical Journal Vol. 1, No. 4330 (Jan. 1, 1944), pp. 8-10
17. *A study of neurosis among repatriated prisoners of war', 17 November 1945, BMJ*
18. ibid

19. ibid
20. The Prisoner of War Mentality: Its Effect After Repatriation by P.H. Neman, D.S.O., M.C., F.R.C.S. BMJ, January 1944
21. ibid
22. ibid
23. *Gloucester Citizen* – Friday 18 July 1947
24. *Belfast Telegraph* – Thursday 17 April 1947
25. *Nottingham Journal* – Thursday 23 January 1947
26. https://archives.friendsqmh.com/1939-59/
27. https://archives.friendsqmh.com/1939-5d
28. https://www.captivememories.org.uk/william-brown
29. *Daily Mirror* – Thursday 28 June 1945
30. *Nottingham Journal* – Saturday 19 February 1949
31. ibid

## Chapter Seven

1. Lieutenant General Percival's letter. The National Archives

# Bibliography

**Barham, Peter**, Forgotten Lunatics of the Great War, Yale University Press

**Bennett, Angela**, The Geneva Convention, The Hidden Origins of the Red Cross, Sutton Publishing

**Bion, Wilfred**, War Memoirs 1917–1919: Second Edition, Routledge

**Bion, Wilfred**, Elements of Psycho-analysis, Routledge

**Bowman, Archibald**, Sonnets From a Prison Camp, Kormendi Press

**Brown, Pam**, Henry Dunant, The Founder of the Red Cross – His Compassion Has Saved Millions, Exley publications

**Dunant, J. Henry,** A Memory of Solferino, Cassell and Company Ltd

**Parker, David,** War Diaries of the First World War

**Parkin, Monty**, Surviving By Magic: The Remarkable Story of Fergus Anckorn, Magician and Survivor of the Thai-Burma Railway

**Peters, John, and Nichol, John**: Tornado Down, Penguin

**Trotter, Wilfred,** Instincts of the Herd in Peace and War, Suzeteo

**Yarnall, John,** Barbed Wire Disease: British and German Prisoners of War, 1914-1919, The History Press

## Websites and online archives

https://encyclopedia.1914-1918-online.net/article/war_psychiatry_and_shell_shock

https://universitystory.gla.ac.uk/ww1-biography/?id=1471

https://ibccdigitalarchive.lincoln.ac.uk/omeka/collections/document/22597

https://www.cofepow.org.uk